NURSING
Student's Guide to
Clinical Success

LORENE PAYNE, EdD, MSN, RN, CNE

The University of Texas
M.D. Anderson Cancer Center
Houston, Texas

610.7307
P346

JONES AND BARTLETT PUBLISHERS
Sudbury, Massachusetts
BOSTON   TORONTO   LONDON   SINGAPORE

World Headquarters

Jones and Bartlett Publishers
40 Tall Pine Drive
Sudbury, MA 01776
978-443-5000
info@jbpub.com
www.jbpub.com

Jones and Bartlett Publishers
Canada
6339 Ormindale Way
Mississauga, Ontario L5V 1J2
Canada

Jones and Bartlett Publishers
International
Barb House, Barb Mews
London W6 7PA
United Kingdom

Jones and Bartlett's books and products are available through most bookstores and online booksellers. To contact Jones and Bartlett Publishers directly, call 800-832-0034, fax 978-443-8000, or visit our website, www.jbpub.com.

Substantial discounts on bulk quantities of Jones and Bartlett's publications are available to corporations, professional associations, and other qualified organizations. For details and specific discount information, contact the special sales department at Jones and Bartlett via the above contact information or send an email to specialsales@jbpub.com.

The authors, editors, and publisher have made every effort to provide accurate information. However, they are not responsible for errors, omissions, or for any outcomes related to the use of the contents of this book and take no responsibility for the use of the products and procedures described. Treatments and side effects described in this book may not be applicable to all people; likewise, some people may require a dose or experience a side effect that is not described herein. Drugs and medical devices are discussed that may have limited availability controlled by the Food and Drug Administration (FDA) for use only in a research study or clinical trial. Research, clinical practice, and government regulations often change the accepted standard in this field. When consideration is being given to use of any drug in the clinical setting, the health care provider or reader is responsible for determining FDA status of the drug, reading the package insert, and reviewing prescribing information for the most up-to-date recommendations on dose, precautions, and contraindications, and determining the appropriate usage for the product. This is especially important in the case of drugs that are new or seldom used.

Production Credits

Publisher: Kevin Sullivan
Acquisitions Editor: Amy Sibley
Associate Editor: Patricia Donnelly
Editorial Assistant: Rachel Shuster
Production Editor: Amanda Clerkin
Marketing Manager: Rebecca Wasley

V.P., Manufacturing and Inventory Control: Therese Connell
Composition: DDC/ASI
Cover Design: Scott Moden
Cover Image Credit: © Carlos Arranz/ShutterStock, Inc.
Printing and Binding: Malloy, Inc.
Cover Printing: Malloy, Inc.

Library of Congress Cataloging-in-Publication Data
Payne, Lorene.
  Nursing student's guide to clinical success / Lorene Payne.
    p. ; cm.
  Includes bibliographical references and index.
  ISBN-13: 978-0-7637-7614-5 (alk. paper)
  ISBN-10: 0-7637-7614-9 (alk. paper)
  1. Nursing—Study and teaching. I. Title.
  [DNLM: 1. Clinical Competence. 2. Education, Nursing. 3. Students, Nursing. WY 18 P346n 2011]
  RT73.P39 2011
  610.73071'1—dc22
                                                        2009033405
6048

Printed in the United States of America
14 13 12 11 10   10 9 8 7 6 5 4 3 2

To all future nurses, my wish and prayer is that you will touch lives gently, expertly, and positively. This book is dedicated to you and the patients you will encounter.

Contents

Acknowledgments

Thank you to all previous patients, whose lives I have touched and who have touched mine. Thanks to my husband for his unwavering support during the writing of this book. I offer gratitude to previous and current colleagues who have shared and continue to share nursing's work, challenges, and blessings. And to the students with whom I have taught and from whom I have learned—thank you!

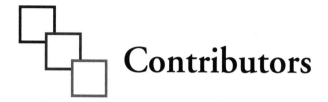 # Contributors

Students benefit from the collective wisdom of many nurses who collaborated on this book.

Dr. Kelly Vandenberg collaborated in the writing of Chapter 10 about the use of simulation as a substitute clinical experience.

I appreciate the participation of all of these contributors: Jean Watson, PhD, RN, AHN-BC, FAAN; Emily Stonebrook, RN; Ann Huntington, BSN, RN; Cherie Howk, PhD, FNP-BC; Mary Ellen Yonushonis, MS, RN, CNE; Sheryl Cornelius, MSN, RN; Lisa Reed, RN; Kiera Noel Thompson, nursing student; Holly Benson, RN; Sylvia Brown, RN; Paige Bentley, BSN, RN; Lauren Shuttlesworth, BSN, RN; Naomi Hayes, RN; Jennifer Donwerth, MSN, RN, ANP-BC, GNP-BC; Rachel Daugherty, MSN, RN; Maureen E. Davis, MSN, RN-BC; Margarita Valdes, MS, RN; Dimitra Loukissa, PhD, RN; Leslie Pafford, RN, PhD, FNP-C; and Alison Carmichael-Bishop, BSN, RN.

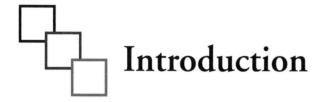

Introduction

I am excited for you as you begin your studies to become a nurse.

Your education will be multifaceted: you will attend classes, take multiple tests, and practice numerous technical skills in lab. Each of these will increase your knowledge and readiness to be a nurse. But the one aspect of your nursing education that pulls it all together is your clinical courses. In clinical courses you will take care of real patients in the actual hospital or clinic setting, applying everything you are learning about.

What a terrific opportunity the clinical courses are!

Clinical experiences are the proving grounds, the places where your learning is more than a test score or completion of a new skill. In clinicals, the humanity of nursing care actually comes through. What you know is partnered with how you care. In clinicals, you become a nurse.

This book provides practical advice and suggestions for making the most of the clinical courses you will have as a nursing student. Please jump right in and get ready to provide the kind of care you would like to receive if you were the patient.

Lorene Payne

Chapter 1

Start from the Heart

"I have always wanted to be a nurse. Even with my dolls as a child, I would bandage them and take care of them."

"I already had a degree and spent the last five years in an industry that is now outsourcing my job. I need a new career!"

"The counselor at high school recommended studying nursing. He says there is a shortage of nurses and I could get a good job that pays well. I've always liked people, so nursing sounds OK."

Welcome to nursing!

Whatever the reason you decided to become a nurse, we need you and welcome you to the profession. Hopefully, you are excited as you begin your nursing education. You are about to embark on quite a journey! Nursing education is more than simply learning facts, although you will certainly add to the many facts you already know. More than that, though, nursing education involves a process of becoming.

You are about to become a nursing professional. Not only will you learn many sciences such as pathology and pharmacology, you will also become part of the culture of nursing. That culture is as much about empathy and advocacy as it is about knowledge. As such, your nursing education will include the human side of things. It is this aspect that elevates the profession and provides an increased benefit to the patients under your care. They are not simply receiving the proper medicine or correct sterile dressing change. They are receiving these interventions from a human being who conveys compassion.

1

Nursing is a profession—the provision of competent technical care—with a human touch. It is also an action word! We take action as we care for people. Your nursing education allows you to practice. You will take care of real people in real nursing settings. This clinical practice enhances the process of you becoming a nurse. Courses which include providing direct patient care are called clinical courses, or clinicals for short.

This is the best type of learning! Working as a student nurse in the clinical setting provides the opportunity to apply what you are hearing in the classroom and seeing in the skills lab. It fosters the type of thinking that is needed to become a nurse. It allows you to practice new skills under the supervision of an experienced nurse. It translates classroom discussions into realities and allows you to ask questions. Clinicals are great!

This book lays the groundwork for success in the clinical courses you will take as a student nurse.

What are Clinicals Like?

Your clinical course will take you into hospitals and other healthcare facilities. You will dress in a nursing uniform, "scrubs," with the colors and/or patch of your college. Part of your uniform will be a stethoscope, watch with a second hand, and white nursing shoes. You are going to look the part and clinicals help you learn to act the part, too!

The State Boards of Nursing in your state regulate how many hours of clinical experience are required. Expect to have 1 or 2 days a week of clinicals each semester you are in nursing school. The State Board also regulates how many student nurses each faculty member can supervise during a clinical day. Typically, each faculty member can have 8–12 students in a clinical group. A clinical instructor may be one of the full-time faculty members or may be a part-time "adjunct" faculty member who handles a clinical group for a shift or two each week.

Obviously, one nurse faculty member cannot be at the side of each of those 8–12 students all of the time during a clinical shift. In a traditional model, student nurses in the clinical group are assigned to a staff nurse, often called the "primary nurse," during the clinical day. The student nurse works with the primary nurse to provide nursing care for a patient or patients. The primary nurse varies from shift to shift as the student is assigned to many areas of the hospital. All of the students of the same clinical group are in the hospital at the same time, and each student rotates through many units, working with many primary nurses. The instructor is always present and checks each student periodically during the shift, directly supervises learning opportunities, facilitates the student's learning and evaluates clinical performance.

Other models of clinical supervision are sometimes used, too. For instance, instead of one instructor supervising 10 students, the State Board may allow a nursing student to be in the hospital for a clinical course when the instructor is not there at all.

Instead, the student is paired with a preceptor for the semester. The preceptor is a staff nurse at the hospital who is recognized for his or her clinical ability.

Under the preceptor model of clinical supervision, the student nurse completes the required number of clinical hours always on the same unit and always with the same preceptor nurse. The student's schedule is determined by the preceptor's schedule. Other students may or may not be in the hospital at the same time. The student nurse is not part of a clinical group, but instead is under the "apprenticeship" of the one preceptor nurse. The faculty member oversees the clinical experience through email contact with the preceptor, face to face meetings and occasional visits to the hospital.

Most programs reserve the preceptor model of clinicals for advanced students who are independent, self-directed workers. The traditional approach of clinical groups with an instructor present during the shift is most common for beginning students. Because of that, most aspects of this book are geared for the traditional clinical course.

Whichever model your college follows for the clinical experience, you will get real experience with real patients in the actual hospital setting. Now that is education!

Nursing as Caring

When you are working in the hospital during clinicals, you will quickly see how much time is spent with patients. Sometimes, the nurse is providing direct care, such as helping the patient walk or eat; sometimes, the nurse is giving medications or dealing with various tubes or dressings. Other times, the nurse will be listening to the patients' concerns, checking them out from head to toe (called assessment) or teaching them and their family what they need to know. Less frequently, the nurse may actually be involved in responding to an emergency and saving a life with immediate interventions.

The unifying themes through this variety of nursing responsibilities are skills and caring. Clinicals provide the environment to practice nursing under supervision.

The hope is that with each patient interaction, the student nurse demonstrates the human side of compassion. For most student nurses, one of the reasons for studying to be a nurse includes wanting to take care of people. Those who practice nursing with this empathetic approach are rewarded every shift. They are rewarded professionally through the difference they make to the patient. They are also rewarded personally because when we are caring for others, we actually become recipients ourselves. You've probably experienced that before, haven't you?

When a family member, friend or neighbor needed something and you provided it, they thanked you for helping, but you actually felt glad for the opportunity to help. That's what compassionate nursing care is like. It is the golden rule in action and reciprocating right back at you.

People at Their Most Vulnerable

One result of people being so sick they require hospitalization, though, is that they are not at their best. Maybe the patient is experiencing pain or is worried about a threat to his or her health. It is possible that he or she is feeling pressured about money concerns or losing his or her job. Maybe the patient had a big surgical procedure during the hospital stay. Each of these circumstances creates anxiety, fear and discomfort in our patients.

A patient who is usually pleasant, happy and easy-going is not likely to seem that way when hospitalized. And the patient whose personality is, shall we say, abrasive in good times will be more difficult to deal with during the stress of a hospital stay. In other words, this is one of those times that may bring out the worst in people.

Family members are concerned, too, and sometimes seem pushy or demanding during their loved one's hospital stay. It is a reality that in most hospitals, members of the family may be present much of the day. For the most part, this is a benefit to the staff and patient, but because of the difficult circumstances of a hospitalization, families may get tired and grumpy, too.

Does this mean that nurses are working all the time with a bunch of mean people, who go around causing problems and being unhappy?! Not at all, but realize that you are not seeing people at their best. You are seeing people at their most vulnerable.

Understanding this allows the student nurse to put comments or difficulties into perspective. It allows us to cultivate an attitude of caring that will help the people in our care make it through these tough times of their hospital stay. It is easier to hear patients' concerns and avoid taking negative comments personally when we appreciate the pressure that our patients and families feel.

Another aspect of hospitalization that makes people feel vulnerable is the loss of independence and privacy. Imagine wearing a "gown" that is all open in the back, being unable to wipe yourself after bathroom activities, enduring strangers gazing at your private areas and wondering if you will recover. All of these common hospital occurrences threaten our patients' sense of well-being.

Because they are so vulnerable and needy, though, another very common human response is gratitude. You are going to experience some humbling expressions of thanks from those you care for. Especially as a student, you have time to listen and to hold their hands both figuratively and literally. Nurses really touch hearts by showing that we care in what we say, how we say it and in all that we do. Patients and families appreciate nurses!

Students at Their Most Vulnerable

Nursing education is not exactly like other college majors. If you are studying finance or history or other degrees, you will go to classes, take tests and complete projects. Studying nursing, you will do all of those things; in addition, you will go to clinicals.

This adds another dimension that leaves the student vulnerable too. As a student nurse, you will expand not just your brain but also your humanity.

You will see situations involving ethical questions. You will be close with life and death. Patients' families and friends will amaze you with examples of the best of human nature, coming through brilliantly to help their loved ones. Other times, you will witness the heartbreak of abandoned patients with no one to care for them. Nursing involves caring for people of every color, age, culture and language and all of the richness—and challenge—entailed in that.

All of these aspects challenge a student nurse to examine individual feelings and values during nursing school. It may be the first time in your life to deal so directly with these very personal, very important issues. Students who are already comfortable in their values and feelings may be challenged by exposure to so many diverse attitudes. Talk to your own family and fellow students when you need to. Draw strength, clarity and direction from your own religious faith and family background. Search for resources such as books or articles that speak to you and help you.

In addition, there is the performance aspect of clinicals where you are actually showing an instructor that you have the ability and understanding of this profession called nursing. Dealing with critical issues and handling yourself in front of the patient and instructor sometimes makes students feel vulnerable. Believe in yourself! The fact that you want to be a nurse, have been chosen from all of the applicants and are applying yourself to your studies testify to your ability to do it. You are ready for the process of becoming a nurse.

Humbling Nature of Intimacy with Strangers

Nursing clinical courses also bring you up close and personal with intimacy, and that intimacy is with strangers. Oh my!

As a student nurse, you are going to be asking people personal questions. Here are just a few examples from among the many, many questions we ask: when was your last bowel movement? Do you leak urine when you cough or laugh? Is the medicine affecting your sex life? When was your last period?

Then there are the times we need to help a person with activities that are usually private: bathing, using the bathroom and cleaning up afterwards, feeding, brushing teeth, etc. Or we are examining the skin for bedsores (called decubitus) which requires looking at all pressure points, including the coccyx. Or we are completing a full head-to-toe assessment invading privacy of all kinds.

How can nurses do that?

We do it as we do all of our nursing care: with compassion and respect. Such a high level of intimacy requires that we exercise that golden rule of handling difficult interactions in a manner we hope others would do with us. Not apologetically. Not without feeling. Not with embarrassment. Not while laughing nervously. We approach all of this with empathy for the patient's feelings and with a straightforward manner that conveys gentle caring and a competence to complete what is needed.

Can you do that? Of course you can—you are becoming a nurse!

Rising to the Call

As you begin this process of becoming a nurse, please open your mind and your heart and take advantage of the real people and real experiences you will have in clinicals. Ask questions. Think. Care. There is much to learn, but much that you already know. You know how to be a caring human being. You know how you would like to be treated. You can put that to use immediately in your clinical shifts. The rest will come with practice and more education.

Example 1-1

The caring side of nursing comes through in the most simple of interactions.

The student nurse was at the nurse's station on the orthopedic floor of a busy hospital looking for a laboratory report. A woman came up to the counter and looked expectantly at the staff. It was obvious that she had a question or needed some help. The student noted that no one else responded to her presence. So, with a smile and looking the woman in the eye, she asked *"Is there something I can do for you?"* The woman smiled with relief. "Yes, thank you. I hate to bother you all. I know nurses are busy. I need. . ."

Example 1-2

After his patient complained of having difficulty sleeping the previous night because of being so cold, the student nurse promised to get her an extra blanket. The shift was almost over and the student was looking forward to getting home, but remembering his promise, took an extra blanket into the patient's room. The patient was ecstatic "You remembered! Oh, thank you so much. Now tonight maybe I can get some sleep. How sweet of you to remember."

Example 1-3

The caring is often directed toward our colleagues.

The student nurse was in a long-term care facility which was filled with many senior citizens with multiple needs. There was an atmosphere of activity and all nursing staff were very busy. One of the nursing assistants came out of a room, shaking her head and mumbling under her breath, "Every time I think I have him cleaned up, he needs cleaning again!" while heading to the clean linens. The student nurse offered to help, "It's always easier with two of us." Sharing the load of a shift is invaluable to building up the team. Another benefit of practicing nursing in this manner: you will always have a hand from others when you need it.

Example 1-4

A valuable reminder is that the nurse–patient interaction is all about the patient, not the nurse.

The student nurse was working with a patient who had suffered a cerebrovascular accident, or stroke, which left her with paralysis of the right side. Feeding her bite by bite took a long time and, to make the patient comfortable, the student nurse began talking. She told the patient about her 3-year-old daughter. The patient asked questions about the child in-between bites of her breakfast. By the time breakfast was over, the patient knew a great deal about the student nurse, but the student nurse knew very little about the patient.

A better approach is to turn questions back to the patient. If, for instance, the patient asks you, "Do you have children?" you can respond with something like, "Yes, I have been blessed with two children. I see cards here on the window sill that came from people who love you! Please tell me about *your* family."

Asking questions about the patient that require more than a simple "yes" or "no" answer are effective in getting the patient talking. These are known as open-ended questions. Think about how you can phrase your questions into an open-ended format. You will find people love to talk about themselves! And you will learn things that help a good nurse provide excellent care. It's all about the patient!

Example 1-5

It is humbling how easily patients allow students to participate in their very personal, important life events.

The student nurse was really looking forward to this particular clinical day—she was going to labor and delivery (L&D)! Her classmates who had already completed their assignment in L&D shared with her how exciting it was to see a baby born. They loved the way the primary nurse helped them know how to support the laboring woman during the process. But best of all, everyone spoke of that awesome moment when the baby actually came screaming out into the world! Wow! Indeed that was how her shift began.

Her day in L&D ended with difficulty, though, as she was reminded of the sobering aspects of the real world: things don't always go well. One young pregnant mom who was carrying twins came in with premature labor and the babies died (called fetal demise). The student nurse chose to help with the babies' postmortem care. Although the little premies did not look totally "normal," she marveled at the little fingers and perfect ears and was surprised that they had wisps of hair on their heads.

Even in this loss, she witnessed how nurses' caring can help a patient.

The nurses cleaned and dressed the little ones in special gowns (volunteers made them for this specific use) and caps. They took pictures and footprints and placed little hospital ID bands on their tiny wrists. The student and the nurses all cried with the mom when she held her babies and told them goodbye. But the nurses were right there and so helpful in this time of almost inconsolable grief.

Example 1-6

Be ready to provide your patient comfort even in potentially embarrassing circumstances.

The student nurse was about 20 years old and was assigned to a postoperative floor. Her patient was in his 30s and had extensive surgery for multiple injuries suffered in a motorcycle accident. The student encouraged him to clean his own face and the upper body parts he could reach, but she was finishing up the lower extremities and perineal area.

As she washed his scrotum and penis, much to his embarrassment, he got an erection. He stammered an apology and actually blushed. Even though the student was initially embarrassed, she didn't want to add to his discomfort, so simply reassured him that it was not a problem, covered him up, and completed the bath without further reference. Her recognition that this incident was simply physiology and not a sexual overture eased her patient's embarrassment.

Example 1-7

Nurses provide care without judging the patient.

A teenage girl who was assaulted at a friend's party came to the emergency center (EC) for attention. The story unfolded that there were no parents or adults present and the teens had been drinking. Her parents met her at the EC and, although relieved she was not more badly injured, were furious with her behavior. As parents, they responded from that perspective.

As the nurse caring for the patient, our perspective is not to lecture or judge the situation. Nor do we approve or make excuses to the parents in a misdirected attempt to "support" the patient. We simply provide the needed nursing care with tenderness and care.

Example 1-8

Many of the most touching examples of nursing's caring come at the end of life.

The patient was in the terminal stages of his disease process and had gone home to die in a comfortable setting, surrounded by his family. The student nurse was assigned to observe a hospice nurse make rounds on her home care patients and they arrived at his home. She was surprised at how upbeat the visit was. The nurse, family and patient smiled and joked and shared stories.

She watched as the hospice nurse assured the patient had adequate pain medication and supervised the wife perform colostomy care perfectly. The wife was worried that he wasn't eating much and the nurse gently reassured her there was no need to push food on him. She was relieved that it was OK to be satisfied with the milkshake he wanted to sip.

The hospice nurse related to the student how the patient had told her on a previous visit, "Don't worry. I have what I need and I am ready. Ain't none of us gonna get out of here alive anyway." Seeing how comfortable and loving the environment was, and how much comfort the family drew from the nurses' visit really made the student proud to be entering such a compassionate profession that had something to offer even in the dying process.

You can see evidence of how very much nursing care is appreciated. Most units have a bulletin board or a countertop or a wall filled with thank you cards from grateful patients and/or family members. Phrases such as, "I don't know how we would have

Nurstoons

by Carl Elbing

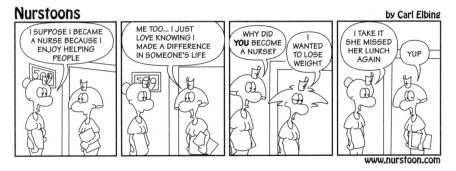

www.nurstoon.com

Figure 1-1   (Courtesy of Carl Elbing, available at http://www.nurstoon.com.)

made it through such a difficult hospitalization without you nurses!" or, "Thank you for taking such good care of my wife. Everyone at the hospital was great—especially the nurses who were truly our angels." or, "My dad was not happy to have to be in the hospital, but the nurses on the cardiac floor really helped. Thanks for making such a stressful time tolerable."

Whatever the reason you came to nursing school—welcome to nursing!

Chapter 2
From Classroom to Clinical

"My friend got into nursing school last year. She is real smart and always got high scores on tests. But she says they spend a lot of shifts in the hospital with patients and it's different than taking a test. I mean, it's the real thing! I hope I can do a good job at it."

"I like people and spent some time as a volunteer in the hospital during high school. But I didn't realize there was so much to do as a nurse. We are learning so many different things. I hope I can keep it all straight when I have a real patient."

"My friend had her first clinicals last semester and said it was so great! Instead of just listening to an instructor talk about diseases and stuff, she said taking care of real people reminded her why she wants to be a nurse."

The goal is to get that license, to add the initials RN after your name, and make a decent living. The ultimate goal is to safely and compassionately take care of people who need your help. To reach these admirable goals, you are in school studying. Classes include pathology, pharmacology, anatomy and physiology and nursing fundamentals, and then the advanced courses. You will learn about disease processes, surgery and medication, and other treatments. You will memorize books worth of facts.

But until you learn to apply what you have studied in the classroom to the patients you take care of in the hospital, you have not met your goals. In this chapter, we will discuss how to cultivate the ability to do just that. Your advantage is that you are already an accomplished student. The proof is that you have been accepted into nursing school. You have an admirable record and have passed tests. You have been chosen from many applicants. This proves, among other things, your mastery of memorization and information.

But in nursing school, mastery of the facts is not enough. It is the place to start, but once you have mastered facts from reading, attending lectures and studying, you will then go to the hospital and take care of patients. Here is where you put what was discussed in the classroom into action in real life.

Applying the Facts

The ideal situation for transferring classroom study into clinical care is to find a patient with the disease process you were studying in class that week. But whether your patient has a diagnosis you have studied or not, here is an approach that allows you to apply the facts to your clinical situation.

Consider what facts you have learned and how you can apply them to this particular patient by asking yourself these questions:

- **What system is involved in the disease process, and what is its normal function?**
- **Because of this system compromise, what will your patient feel? In other words, what symptoms do you expect to find in your patient?**
- **Because of these symptoms, what nursing care measures can make your patient more comfortable and/or help them heal?**
- **What are the usual medical treatments for this problem?**
- **Can this pathology be cured? Improved? Or will it be chronic?**
- **How can you tell if the interventions are working?**

Where can you get the answers to these questions if you haven't yet studied the disease? There are many resources: your clinical instructor, the staff nurse taking care of the patient, the hospital's intranet, or you may refer to reference books or a PDA program of diseases. The patient will hopefully know many of the answers, too. Practice interviewing skills to find out what they know, how much they understand and what the doctor has told them. They may have a beginning answer for many of the questions listed above from which you can verify and expand.

Recognizing How It Fits

This sounds like a lot to understand. After all, you are just beginning your education. Taking it one step at a time though, you can see how straightforward it really is. We'll answer each of the questions for a **simple infected wound**.

- **What system is involved in the disease process, and what is its normal function?** The skin is involved (medically this is referred to as the integumentary system). Intact skin is a barrier to disease-causing germs (pathogens) and also helps control fluid balance and temperature. We could also say the body's defense system is involved in trying to clear the infection. The circulating white blood cells (WBCs) and the lymph system attack pathogens to clear infections.
- **Because of this system compromise, what symptoms do you expect to find in your patient?** At the wound site, you expect to see an open wound with redness, swelling and maybe drainage. All of these symptoms show that the body is mobilizing to fight the invading pathogens. From the body defense response, expect to see a fever and an increase in the infection fighting cells (an increased WBC). Also from the body's reaction, the patient may feel low in energy (lethargic), have generalized aches or pain localized to the infected area.
- **Because of these symptoms, what nursing care measures can make your patient more comfortable and/or help them heal?** The following measures might help: cleaning and dressing the wound, taking a culture and sensitivity (a sample of the drainage from the wound so the lab can identify the germ causing the infection and which antibiotic can kill the germ), washing hands well after touching the wound or dressings, encouraging the patient to drink fluids, providing nutritious food that promotes healing, keeping the room cool if they have a fever, providing a cool washcloth for comfort and to decrease fever, teaching them the proper way to take antibiotics, teaching them infection control measures, and allowing them to rest.
- **What are the usual medical treatments for this problem?** Administering antibiotics to fight the infection, giving medication to bring down the fever if it gets too high and mild pain relievers as needed. Expect contact precautions (hand washing, use of gloves when coming in contact with soiled dressings and proper disposal of dressings). For severely infected wounds, surgical or topical debridement (cleaning out of the dead tissue) may be needed. If there are other medical conditions that interfere with healing (like diabetes or poor wound circulation), those conditions need to be brought under control, too.
- **Can this pathology be cured?** Yes, a wound infection should be cleared and a scar should grow over the healed area if the patient does not have other medical complications.

- **How can you tell if the interventions are working?** If the comfort measures work, the patient will feel better; if the antibiotics work, the signs of infection will decrease within a day or two of beginning antibiotics, and the lab values of the infection-fighting cells will decrease as the infection is brought under control; if the antipyretic medications (to take down the fever) work, the temperature will return to normal; if the pain medications work, the pain will decrease; if your hand washing technique is good, the infection will not spread; if your teaching is good, the patient will comply with the medical plan.

See how straightforward it is? Of course, for more complicated disease processes the answers are more complex. But it all boils down to these simple aspects. Asking these questions takes the facts you have studied and applies them to your patient. Then you can put this into action in the hospital as you care for your patient and your learning continues.

In the infected wound example, the classroom lecture would have discussed the layers of skin, the stages of wound healing, the types of WBCs that respond to the infection, etc. Pharmacology class would have provided information about different classes of antibiotics and methods of administering them. Skills lab would have shown you how to collect a specimen for culture and sensitivity. Nursing fundamentals will address hand washing and protective equipment (gloves, etc.). In more advanced classes, the nursing student will add more information about infections and the body's response. For instance, you will find that diabetes or other diseases interfere with healing and will learn about the specific laboratory tests that will provide information to direct and evaluate care.

Another part of the curriculum will cover patient teaching. The student nurse will learn to consider assessing first what the patient knows, barriers to learning, how to present information, etc. Applying patient education to the infected wound example, the student nurse will recognize that the patient needs to wash their hands, eat adequate protein and take their medication as ordered. You will come to understand that the patient needs to clearly see *why* it is important to take medications or eat certain foods (or avoid others) and a myriad of other self-care practices that require a change in lifestyle. The better job nurses do teaching our patients, the more compliant they are and better outcomes are seen. When patients understand why and how specific measures help them, they usually want to embrace the things that will help them heal.

You will be tested in the classroom on these types of facts. In the clinical setting, you relate these to what you see in your patient and what you do because of it. It is in this setting that you can truly demonstrate that you are on your way to becoming a nurse. Applying what you know from the classroom to what your patients need is the mark of critical thinking or clinical reasoning and a huge step towards realizing your goals.

Let's take another common medical problem and approach it using this format to help direct our thinking and apply the facts we know to the patient problems we are seeing. This time we will focus on congestive heart failure (CHF). CHF is one of the most common admitting diagnoses, so you can expect to see it in the hospital.

- **What system is involved in the disease process, and what is its normal function?** The cardiovascular system is involved in CHF. Usually, the heart acts like a pump and receives blood from the body, sends it to the lungs for oxygenation and then sends it to the body. In CHF, the heart muscle (myocardium) is not efficiently pumping blood around the body because the cardiac muscles themselves are weak.
- **Because of this system compromise, what will your patient feel? In other words, what symptoms do you expect to find in your patient?** When the blood is not pumped efficiently, it may back up into the lungs so the patient may feel short of breath; we may actually hear fluid at the bases of the lungs when we put a stethoscope to the back. The sound heard in the lungs is called "crackles" and the problem it shows is pulmonary edema. The patient will fatigue easily because of poor oxygenation (which can be measured by a pulse oximeter machine) and may not be able to handle all of their self-care activities. There may be swelling of the ankles (called pedal edema) as the poorly circulating blood fluids leak out into the dependant tissues. Blood pressure may fall because of the weak pumping action. Kidneys don't work as well when the blood pressure is low, so urine output may decrease and fluid may build up in the body resulting in weight gain. More than 2 pounds of weight gain in 24 hours, or 5 pounds in a week, is usually considered fluid gain.
- **Because of these symptoms, what nursing care measures can make your patient more comfortable and/or help them heal?** You can give oxygen, allow rest periods between activities, weigh the patient daily and report to the physician any significant weight gain, teach the patient about their medications and self-care measures, teach about limiting salt in the diet to minimize fluid retention, encourage patient to elevate feet if pedal edema is present, assist with cardiac rehabilitation as possible (i.e., patient exercises to tolerance under supervision and builds cardiac muscle strength), administer medications and assess for their effects.
- **What are the usual medical treatments for this problem?** Conservative treatment is used most often: medications to improve the strength of the heart muscle (digitalis), medication to encourage the body to urinate out extra fluid (diuretics), medication to replace other components excreted in the urine because of the diuretics (i.e., potassium), tests to monitor the heart function (blood tests and cardiac function tests) and monitored exercise to improve

myocardial strength. Extreme treatment would be implanting a mechanical pump or heart transplant surgery.

- **Can this pathology be cured? Improved? Or will it be chronic?** Unless the heart muscle is weak because of a reversible condition, it cannot be cured. Most heart failure will be chronic and over the years will progressively worsen. If the patient complies with the treatment (taking medications, limiting salt and getting exercise), then he or she can have improved myocardial strength and often can continue to be independent in their daily activities for years. Surgery is used in extreme cases. Either a mechanical pump can be implanted to assist the weak heart or a replacement heart may be transplanted. These surgical interventions may be considered cures for the heart failure, but these treatments themselves create new problems.

- **How can you tell if the interventions are working?** Improved vital signs and activity tolerance, decrease in pulmonary and pedal edema and loss of fluid weight.

You can see by these two examples that applying the classroom information about pathology and disease as you work with your patient really allows you to "see" the effects, treatment and outcomes and understand why the things you see happen. When you approach clinical care with this framework in mind, answering these questions and incorporating nursing care to assist your patient, nursing is interesting and makes quite a difference in the quality of life and often the actual outcome for your patient. This approach can begin right inside the classroom if you require yourself to put the information in context of patient care. Let's call it "Build a Patient."

Build a Patient

Building a patient during classroom activities means that, as the lecture and readings impart facts about pathology, nursing care and medical care, the student nurse actively translates these pieces of information into a scenario that creates a fictional patient. The information is not simply memorized into lists of symptoms or words detailing pathophysiology. Instead, the facts are incorporated into their impact on a human being. The student is building a theoretical patient as the new material is learned.

Using the question set offered at the beginning of this chapter can direct study and help to build the patient. Discussing this in study groups also assists. Some students benefit from actually drawing a picture of what the assessment of a patient with these symptoms would show. Others have created an outline drawing of a person (the

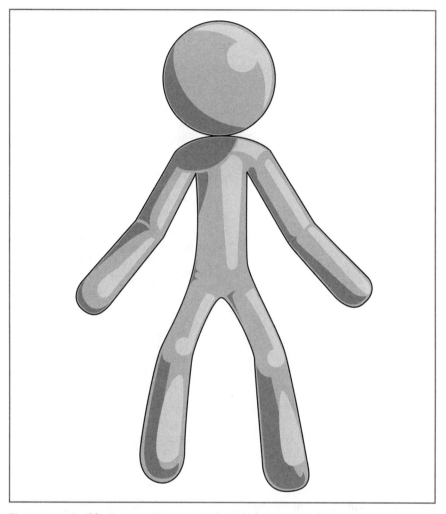

Figure 2-1   Build a Patient. Create a simple stick figure—you don't have to be an artist!

patient) and attached sticky notes of the assessment findings on the appropriate body part.

Of course, not every patient with a specific diagnosis will actually manifest all of the possible symptoms of that disease, but picturing all that is possible prepares the student for anything. Once you have a picture of a patient with a specific disease, next picture what the nurse can do about it. Let's call this "Build a Nurse."

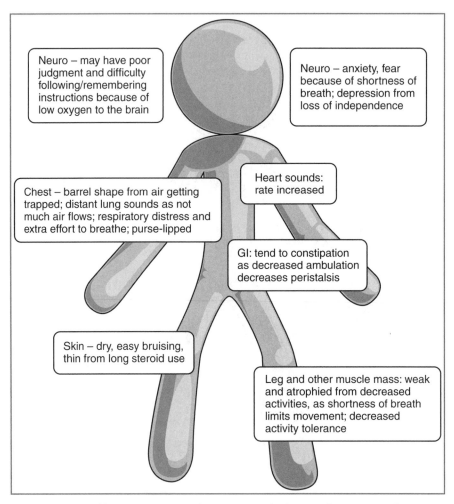

Neuro – may have poor judgment and difficulty following/remembering instructions because of low oxygen to the brain

Neuro – anxiety, fear because of shortness of breath; depression from loss of independence

Chest – barrel shape from air getting trapped; distant lung sounds as not much air flows; respiratory distress and extra effort to breathe; purse-lipped

Heart sounds: rate increased

GI: tend to constipation as decreased ambulation decreases peristalsis

Skin – dry, easy bruising, thin from long steroid use

Leg and other muscle mass: weak and atrophied from decreased activities, as shortness of breath limits movement; decreased activity tolerance

Figure 2-2   Build a Patient. Example: patient with chronic obstructive pulmonary disease.

Build a Nurse

Once the fictitious patient has been built and the expected assessment findings pictured, turn your attention to what the nurse can do to help. Building the nurse to address the patient findings requires you to actively consider helpful nursing interventions. Allow yourself to derive these actions directly from what you pictured in Build a Patient. When you study and prepare in this manner, you can understand why certain interventions are taken rather than just memorizing them.

Some of the actions you will build into your nurse concern the medical tests and/or treatments for the pathology. For instance, in the example of an infection, antibiotics will be ordered. But don't limit yourself to simply the administration of the medications. There are almost always considerations about those medications: does the patient have allergies that contradict the drug? Does the drug conflict with any current medications the patient is on? What is the best route to administer the drug? If intravenous (IV) administration is optimal, provide the appropriate access if the patient does not already have an IV. Are there interactions with food or other medications that must be considered? If the patient is to continue the medication, what self-administration instructions are necessary? Are there laboratory tests to watch that indicate outcome of the drug or that show potential negative side effects?

Building a nurse to help your patient also requires that you look at any procedures or tests your patient may undergo and what role the nurse may play in them: is there preparation before the test? What instruction does the patient require? Must the patient fast? Determine the specifics about the test or procedure so the patient clearly knows what to expect: will the doctor perform the test at the bedside? Or does the patient go to a different department? How long does the procedure take? Will the patient be lying on a cold hard table or be in an enclosure? After the test is done, how long before the results are known? And finally, what exactly can be determined from the test?

Can you see how simply knowing that specific tests are to be done is not good enough? You must take the classroom information beyond the facts and visualize how they actually affect your patient and what you as a nurse can do to help. Take your Build a Nurse exercise beyond the medical responses, too. Nurses do more than simply administer medications or prepare patients for tests.

Much of what the nurse offers is personal human caring. We began this book with a tribute to the human side of nursing. You apply this in innumerable simple ways: smiling as you perform your nursing tasks, listening to the patient's concerns and genuinely caring, patting them on the shoulder when they need encouragement, going out of your way to assist them in contacting their families, the list hopefully goes on and on. Remember this very important aspect of your care as you Build a Nurse: treating our patients as we would want our loved ones treated is the perfect approach.

Also build in the assessments to make for this specific patient problem. Hopefully, you will avoid simply listing things that you learned in the classroom: monitor vital signs, monitor temperature, assess for fluid balance, etc. Go above that and picture what exactly you will watch for. For instance with the CHF patient mentioned earlier, instead of saying "monitor fluid volume," think about what exactly you will see if the person is having fluid volume problems. The weight will increase since water has weight. So build in to your nurse "monitor daily weights for gain more than 2 pounds in 24 hours or more than 5 pounds in a week." That is much clearer and shows you know how to apply what you learned about fluid volume problems to an actual patient situation.

Another aspect of building a nurse is to consider what information your patient needs you to teach. Again, be specific. Stating that the nurse will teach about medications is correct. But detailing what teaching points need to be covered takes your Build a Nurse to a deeper level. For instance, the patient mentioned earlier with CHF will take a heart muscle strengthening medicine, like digoxin. But don't simply Build a Nurse to instruct in digoxin self-administration. Look it up and detail exactly what to teach: self-pulse check, holding the digoxin if the pulse is below 60, and report any signs of digitalis toxicity such as nausea, slow pulse, or visual changes like halos around objects or blind spots. As you study and Build the Nurse, your understanding will increase with this extra attention to detailing specifics.

Building a nurse will also include aspects of the type of diet the patient needs. Does the pathology require them to change their diet? For instance, the CHF patient we used earlier in this chapter would likely be expected to limit salt intake. Why? Remember this patient is at risk for fluid volume overload. Salt attracts water, so if salt is unrestricted it will add to the fluid held in the body and worsen the fluid volume overload. Limiting salt will limit fluid retention and give the heart less circulating volume to handle. When you Build a Nurse regarding salt restriction, include what you will teach your patient and why this intervention and instruction helps the patient's condition.

Activity is another area of nursing care to consider as you Build a Nurse. Some disease processes require more rest for the patient to recover. For instance, if the patient is pregnant and threatening to lose the baby early, bedrest will take the weight and pressure of the full uterus off the cervix and might prolong the pregnancy to term. Or if there has been an orthopedic injury, rest is often needed to allow healing.

On the other hand, often the nurse's job is to encourage activity to improve muscular strength and conditioning or to decrease the chances of complications from inactivity. After a cerebrovascular accident (CVA, commonly called a stroke), the patient needs to be encouraged to move around and use gross motor muscle groups. Other conditions benefit from activity, too, and the nurse needs to recognize them and act accordingly.

The Build a Nurse exercise will also incorporate nursing care you learned in nursing fundamentals. An entire group of nursing interventions is standard for our patients who have limitations in their mobility. This would include, for instance, people who cannot walk well because of weakness or restrictions in their movement, whether these are short-term or chronic limitations. The reason nurses treat these patients in special ways is because the limitation puts the patient at risk for many complications.

Think of what happens to different body systems when the patient is in bed more than usual:

- Skin—pressure of body weight on bony points (for instance the tailbone, heels, etc.) pushes blood out of capillary beds and deprives the tissue of nourishment and oxygen. What is the possible result? Bedsores (called decubiti) can form and are very hard to heal. The nursing action that prevents this: change the patient's position every 2 hours and keep the skin clean and dry. Build this into your nursing plan.
- Cardiovascular—less patient movement results in sluggish blood flow. Sluggish blood flow results in increased risk for clots forming (this usually happens in the legs). When clots form in a vessel, they may break off and float around in the blood stream (called an embolus) until they reach a vessel too small to let them pass. This causes a total blockage of blood flow and whatever tissue is supposed to be fed by that vessel will die. (If the clot blocks a heart artery it results in a heart attack, called a myocardial infarction; in the brain, it creates a CVA). The nursing action to help prevent this: have the patient move their feet and legs around every 2 hours even if it is simply moving them in bed, apply compression on the legs to direct the blood flow into deeper veins that don't clot as easily (may be simply elastic stockings or leg wrappings that are pumped and released by a motorized control called sequential compression devices [SCDs]) and sometimes medications are ordered that slow the clotting process.
- Respiratory—the mucus in the lungs tends to settle by gravity when someone lies down. Also, the lungs are not expanded well and the small alveoli at the terminal branches may collapse as a result. These effects leave the immobile patient more at risk for pneumonia, which is infection in the lungs, and also for atelectasis, which is collapse of the alveoli. The nursing action to reduce this risk: have the patient with decreased mobility breathe deeply and force a cough every 2 hours, or use an incentive spirometer provided by the respiratory therapy department, and change position every 2 hours.
- Psychosocial—Patients who are limited in their mobility are often depressed by their dependency on nursing staff for personal care assistance, especially if this represents a change in their usual abilities and/or is likely to become a permanent change. Just think how you would feel if you were normally independent in all of your daily care and suddenly cannot get out of bed and are forced to use a bedpan or cannot wipe yourself after a bowel movement. It is often demoralizing. Worse yet, if this is a condition that is expected to become chronic, it is something the patient must learn to live with. Nursing interventions to help: practicing human compassion as you assist people, respecting their humanity, gently tending to their needs, masking any negative response to unpleasant odors, reminding patients that you are happy for the opportunity to care for them, having them recognize that they would care for you if positions were reversed and if the mobility restriction is to be short-term, the nurse can remind them of that fact.

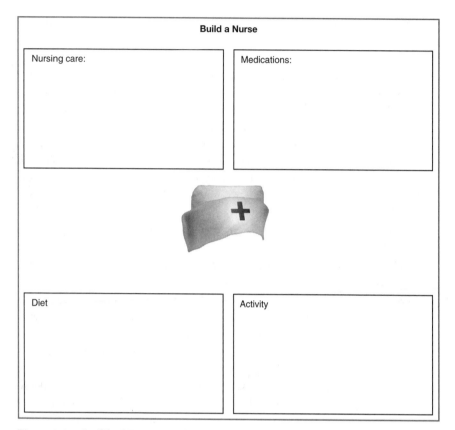

Figure 2-3   Build a Nurse. Here's one way to do this exercise.

- Gastrointestinal—When a body does not move around as much as usual, intestinal peristalsis slows down. This may result in constipation, and in severe cases, it can lead to intestinal obstruction. Nursing interventions to reduce the risk: encourage ambulation as much as possible, administer stool softeners, assure that bowel movement frequency and character is documented daily to prevent excessive delay in evacuation of stool, encourage the patient to take enough fluid each day so that the urine is almost clear as this will keep the stool softer and allow it to pass more easily and administer laxatives or enemas as needed.

As you consider all of these very important nursing interventions to minimize the complications of limited mobility, it is hopefully encouraging to see how much impact good nursing care can have on the outcomes for our patient. When you add these final touches to your Build a Nurse exercise, you will have an excellent picture

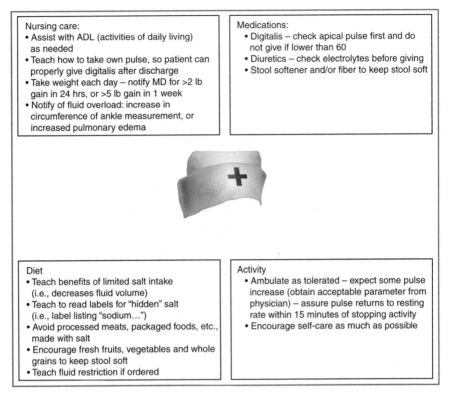

Nursing care:
- Assist with ADL (activities of daily living) as needed
- Teach how to take own pulse, so patient can properly give digitalis after discharge
- Take weight each day – notify MD for >2 lb gain in 24 hrs, or >5 lb gain in 1 week
- Notify of fluid overload: increase in circumference of ankle measurement, or increased pulmonary edema

Medications:
- Digitalis – check apical pulse first and do not give if lower than 60
- Diuretics – check electrolytes before giving
- Stool softener and/or fiber to keep stool soft

Diet
- Teach benefits of limited salt intake (i.e., decreases fluid volume)
- Teach to read labels for "hidden" salt (i.e., label listing "sodium...")
- Avoid processed meats, packaged foods, etc., made with salt
- Encourage fresh fruits, vegetables and whole grains to keep stool soft
- Teach fluid restriction if ordered

Activity
- Ambulate as tolerated – expect some pulse increase (obtain acceptable parameter from physician) – assure pulse returns to resting rate within 15 minutes of stopping activity
- Encourage self-care as much as possible

Figure 2-4   Build a Nurse. Filled out for the patient with CHF referenced earlier.

of the exact care your patient needs from you during your shift. Additionally, you will understand why these interventions are so important and how they benefit your patient. You will make such a difference in your patients' hospital stay!

This concept of applying the information learned in the classroom to the patient in the hospital is crucial to becoming a nurse. Nursing is not a profession in which formulas can simply be memorized and applied. It is not similar to creating a favorite dish by following a recipe. Everyday, with every patient, a good nurse is actively thinking about the individual assessment findings and what they disclose about the patient, their needs and progress. This makes it both more challenging and more rewarding.

Individualizing care makes nursing effective. Student nurses cultivate patient individualization by actively considering how the information they have been studying in the classroom applies to the specific patient in their care. Then, they take that planning and study into the hospital as they assess the real patient and recognize what is needed for that particular patient. When you come to this point, you are becoming a nurse.

Example 2-1

Your patient is 58 years old and had a herniated disc in the lumbar spine. He underwent a laminectomy of L4–L5 2 days ago. He has a dry dressing on the lumbar area of his back and complains of pain at a level of 6 out of 10. Use the guiding questions from the beginning of the chapter:

- **What system is involved in the disease process, and what is its normal function?** A laminectomy is a surgery on the spine, usually to repair a herniated disc, so it is part of the musculoskeletal system. Remember that this system normally provides support and motion for the body. The spine specifically allows for flexibility in the back and provides a passageway for the spinal cord and an exit way for the peripheral nerves. The nervous system is also involved, as the breakdown in the cushion substance between the vertebrae causes the bone to press on the nerve. This is what causes the pain.

- **Because of this system compromise, what will your patient feel? In other words, what symptoms do you expect to find in your patient?** When the musculoskeletal system is compromised, it may limit the person's movement. When the spine is involved, since it carries nerves, pain and/or altered sensations (tingling, numbness) may be expected. So the patient with spinal pathology likely will experience pain with movement, especially movements that require flexibility of or work by the spine (getting up from a lying down position or lifting objects).

- **Because of these symptoms, what nursing care measures can make your patient more comfortable and/or help them heal?** Teaching, demonstrating and assuring the patient uses proper body mechanics is crucial to comfort, function and to minimize the chance of reinjury to the spine, administering pain medication and other pain control measures, helping with daily living activities and movements that may be difficult, providing any equipment that will help movement, dressing care for the surgical site and recognizing that a person who is not moving around as much as usual (nurses call this limited mobility) could get pneumonia, constipation, skin sores (called decubiti) and clots in the legs are some measures that might help the patient. Some interventions nurses encourage to prevent complications of immobility include breathing deeply every few hours, walking around as much as tolerated and drinking enough fluids so that the urine is almost clear.

- **What are the usual medical treatments for this problem?** The laminectomy surgery was the treatment your patient received for the herniated disc. Look at your anatomy and physiology book and you will remember how the vertebrae are separated by a cushioned substance. When that rips and bulges out, it cannot cushion properly and the nerves are pinched, resulting in pain. The surgery cleans up the bulging material and stabilizes the spine again by surgically fixing the vertebrae around the herniation.

Pain medications will be used postoperatively. Other healthcare workers teach the patient exercises to improve strength and safety in daily movements. Physical therapy works more with gross motor movements such as walking and transfer; occupational therapy works more with what is called activities of daily living such as bathing and dressing, among other things. Nurses coordinate with the therapists and help the patients follow the exercises and use any equipment.

- **Can this pathology be cured? Improved? Or will it be chronic?** If all goes well, the surgery is a cure for the herniated disc. However, often a person originally experiences a herniated disc because of poor body mechanics and habits. If they do not make changes in their daily movements, they are at higher risk for suffering another herniation.

- **How can you tell if the interventions are working?** The nurse monitors to ensure postoperative pain is controlled, the surgical site heals without infection and the patient can demonstrate the proper way of getting out of bed (log-rolling technique) and other body movements (e.g., avoiding bending at the waist, avoiding twisting, lifting with the strong muscles in the legs instead of the back).

Example 2-2

Here is an example of a student who always scored high on tests in the lecture courses during nursing school but did not show the ability to apply what she learned to her actual patients in the hospital.

The patient had an infected wound and was on contact precautions. During the Nursing Fundamentals course, the student had learned what contact precautions required and in what patient circumstances they were used. Contact precautions are used when the patient has an infection that could be communicated to someone else who touches the infection source. For this patient, it was an infected wound.

The nursing student had answered the test questions properly, passed the written exam and had been able to don the protective gear in skills lab. Yet in the hospital when she was preparing to administer morning medications to the patient, she entered the room without a gown, checked the apical pulse using her own stethoscope and handed the medications to the patient without wearing gloves.

Each of these actions was a violation of contact precautions, yet she did not recognize it. Her attention was focused on the "higher" skill of medication administration to the point that she totally forgot to apply the isolation precautions.

The instructor stopped her from leaving the room after administering the medication and asked her what she had forgotten to do. Even with this prompting, she could not identify the requirements of contact isolation. She was showing an inability to apply in the hospital what she had learned in the classroom. As a result, she was endangering her patients and herself.

Example 2-3

Happily, there are examples where the student does apply theory to practice.

The student was caring for a patient who had been admitted to the hospital repeatedly with out-of-control blood sugar. She was an insulin-dependant diabetic. Hospital staff believed that the patient was not compliant with her diabetic self-care. Staff assumed that the patient was not eating properly, not checking her blood sugar or taking the insulin as ordered.

In class, the student nurse had studied the pathology of diabetes and learned that the pancreas was not producing insulin. She knew that foods eaten are broken down into sugars and circulated through the bloodstream for the body to use. Insulin takes the sugars out of the bloodstream and into the cells for use. When the body does not produce insulin, the patient experiences two basic problems: the sugars rise in the bloodstream (which is destructive to the brain and to small capillary beds throughout the body) and the cells starve because they can't get the sugars inside the cell to produce energy.

The student nurse had studied in class how the patient needs to replace the insulin not produced by the body with an injection of insulin. Some other requirements for diabetic control at home: checking the blood sugar (with a glucometer) using a fingerstick drop of blood to see how well controlled the blood sugar is and eating properly.

Instead of presuming that the patient had simply decided not to follow proper diabetic self-management, the student nurse had a conversation to assess what the patient understood and what practices she was following. From this assessment, the student discovered the patient seemed to have good understanding of diabetes control. So she asked the patient's daughter to bring into the hospital the patient's own glucometer. By checking the readings against the hospital equipment, the student discovered that the patient's glucometer was not registering accurately. The patient did not have the information she needed to control her blood sugar.

The student's willingness to search for an explanation instead of assuming noncompliance, and because she understood how to apply the theory of diabetic control into an actual patient situation, and because she applied what she learned about the Nursing Process beginning with assessment this student may have saved the patient from future hospitalizations. She truly was an effective nurse that day.

Example 2-4

Another way that a student nurse can demonstrate applying what was learned in the classroom to the hospital clinical work is through discussions with the instructor. Be sure to explain what you understand about your patient. Students who are naturally quiet and don't voice what they are thinking out loud sometimes have difficulty showing that they understand and are applying what they know. Make a conscious effort to verbalize what you know and what you are wondering. Often, your questions reveal as much as other comments or observations and may lead you to learn even more.

One student explained to the clinical instructor that she had a patient with a brain tumor. She understood that it was a cancerous growth in the brain and needed to receive chemotherapy, but that the membrane surrounding the brain limited what could penetrate (this is called the blood-brain barrier). So she asked how the chemotherapy was going to reach the tumor. This question was excellent and indicated that she was applying her anatomy and physiology, pathology and pharmacology to her patient.

After the instructor and student checked the chart and spoke with the patient, it was recognized that this patient was to undergo implantation of a cerebral reservoir. Neither the student nor the instructor had worked with one before, so both did some research. It became a journey of discovery and when the information was understood, the student shared it with the clinical group in postconference (see Chapter 9). The reservoir would be implanted in the brain, filled with the chemotherapy drug and would gradually pump out small amounts right near the tumor. What a wonderful example of taking what you know from the classroom, applying it to your patient and going beyond it to learn even more.

Chapter 3
Take Charge— Managing a Shift

The first clinical shift the student nurse looked the part: clean scrubs, shiny stethoscope around his neck, and shoulder patch announcing school affiliation. But his stomach churned with the question: "Where do I start?"

Two hours into the shift, the student moaned: "I feel like I haven't gotten anything done! My patients wanted to sleep this morning, so I can't bother them until later."

The student nurse complained to her instructor: "My primary nurse suggested I follow her around so I could get the idea of what to do. Now the shift is almost over, and I haven't really done anything!"

Getting Off to the Right Start

One of the biggest challenges for the student nurse is figuring out how to get organized. Each hospital or facility has its own routines, the patients' doctors have specific written orders, each nursing instructor has slightly different expectations and each student comes from a unique background. So is there a way a student nurse can approach a shift and master it? YES!!

Your clinical instructor may have suggestions for you and will help you individualize the recommendations in this chapter to your facility and your nursing program. But the ideas presented here will help you get started. The first part of the shift sets up how smoothly the rest of the shift proceeds, so get a good start!

Picking Good Patients

Some nursing programs require student nurses to go to the hospital the evening before a clinical day and choose their patient(s) for the clinical day. That allows the student to know ahead of time what diagnosis the patient has. In this case, students are expected to prepare a plan for their nursing care the next day. Not all programs require this preclinical planning; and working nurses of course do not come in before a scheduled shift to find out about the patients, so you may not know your patients until the morning you arrive for shift.

Whether you go the evening before or pick patients the morning of, getting the "right" patient helps you cement your learning. If the patient's clinical situation is too complex for you, it will be difficult to make sense of what you are assessing or what interventions to take. Yet, if the patient is too "easy," you will not be challenged to learn, or if you choose the same type of patient each shift because you are comfortable with that type of nursing care, then you are cheated out of advancing.

To help you know what type of patient is appropriate, ask your clinical instructor. You will be given guidelines that correlate with your level of knowledge and with what you are studying in class and skills lab. Most nursing programs begin with basic fundamental care. Included are interventions such as helping a patient with a bath, making a bed (you will even learn how to make a bed with a patient still in it!), assisting them in dressing, shaving and brushing their teeth, etc. These cares are known as Activities of Daily Living (ADL).

Since this is where basic nursing care begins, picking a patient who needs this type of help is a good place to start. Such patients are known as "total care" patients, meaning they need help with all of their ADL. Let your primary nurse know that you need a total care patient. Staff nurses appreciate student nurses' help with total care patients because of the time demands to provide everything for such patients. They will be relieved that you are taking care of the patient!

However, as you progress in your studies, you will take other types of patients and would *not* want a patient who demanded all of your time. Another part of advancing in your studies involves taking more than one patient. When you are ready to take multiple patients, it would be difficult to provide for them all if one or two are total care: there would not be enough time to get it all done. So, later on, you will not want a total care patient but at first this type of patient is perfect.

Remember, before your shift begins, ask your clinical instructor about the type and number of patients you will be expected to care for. Also consider what disease processes you have been covering in class and what skills you have been learning in lab. Share this information with your primary nurse; then you are ready to pick your patient(s). With this in mind, listen to report at the beginning of the shift to hear which patients are on the unit.

The standard for nursing care is that the off-going shift (the nurses who cared for the patients all night before you came that morning) gives report to the oncoming shift (see Chapter 5). Based on this report, you will have a quick picture of your assigned patient(s). You will be told the patient's diagnosis and given an update on their status. You will know what tubes and drains are in place and have a good picture of their needs. Use this report to get started with your patient.

Complementing this oral report from the nurses is some form of written summary you can refer to. It may be a computer printout of the patients on the floor, or it may be individual cards (called a Kardex) for each patient. Whatever format is used in your facility, you will get something in writing about the patients. Use this to take notes about the verbal report you hear and from it pick an appropriate patient.

Additionally, you will have a "primary nurse" or "preceptor nurse" (different programs use different terminology) to work with during the shift. One clinical instructor has many students to supervise during a clinical shift and is not at your side during the whole day. So the student shares the actual care of the patient with the staff nurse who is assigned that patient; this is what is meant by the primary nurse. Before or after receiving report, confer briefly with your primary nurse. The importance of the primary nurse cannot be overemphasized. Be nice to this nurse! You will need his or her support, help and encouragement going through the shift. From this nurse you will learn a tremendous amount, so cultivate an attitude of gratitude from the beginning of the shift.

Assure that the nurse clearly understands the level of your nursing education, aspects of patient care you will take care of and which aspects the staff nurse needs to do. For instance, first semester students may not give medications or may only give some of the scheduled medications. Communicate well what you can and cannot do! Clearly specify if you are going to write in the chart or if the staff nurse will complete the charting. Good communication is essential for safe patient care and to assure there are no mistakes simply because the nurse did not know what the student was or was not going to complete.

One of the mistakes students often make is to spend excessive time in the chart at the beginning of the shift. After receiving report, they head for the patient's chart and start reading, trying to know it all before seeing the patients. This approach is not only unnecessary but also dangerous! Your responsibility begins at the beginning of the shift—not 2 hours later after you have read the entire chart. So, after hearing report, taking notes on your worksheet and talking to your primary nurse, go and assess your patient(s).

Reviewing the beginning of the clinical shift: find your primary nurse and confer with him or her, listen to report, and take notes and then go to your patient(s) room. All of this happens within the first hour of your shift!

Meeting Your Patient(s)

Remember: the patient is why you are becoming a nurse! Although some student nurses are nervous at first, keeping positive and open-minded helps when meeting patients. Knocking on the door, even if it is open, is a respectful way to begin a first greeting. It is especially important since you will likely be waking them up. Most nursing schools place student nurses on day shift beginning around seven in the morning, so as you enter the room, your patient may be asleep or just waking up.

Because of the early hour, your patient's first response, even before you introduce yourself, may be to ask for more time to sleep. Many students immediately apologize and back out of the room to comply. Resist this temptation! Remember, you are responsible for the patient's condition and must evaluate them briefly as you begin the shift. How would you know if they are bleeding, confused or in need if you did not check it out? Nurses call this an assessment. The assessment must be done first thing on the shift.

So, if your patient rolls over and pulls the covers up begging for more sleep, be prepared to empathize with them, yet push for cooperation. You may say something such as, "Hospitals aren't the best places for sleep, are they? I can let you snuggle back in bed soon, but first we need to check you out. It's morning and the new shift is starting." Then begin a quick introduction.

The introduction is important as it sets the stage for your work with the patient. Some students rehearse what they want to say, others play it by ear. Go with your own comfort level, but include in that first introduction your name and the fact that you are a student. Something like: "Hi. Mr. Jones, my name is Laurie. I'm in my first year of nursing school, and I'll be helping to take care of you today." It's best to be short, sweet and confident.

Most patients are amazingly willing to allow student involvement with their care, but some do not want students. The patient has the right to refuse. Let your instructor know immediately if the patient refuses you. A good instructor may sometimes be able to enhance your introduction, and the patient may agree to accept a student after all. If not, involving your instructor quickly verifies this fact. It also allows time to get another patient.

Many hospitals have a white board in each patient room. Writing your name and the primary nurse's name on the board in the patient's room helps the patient to know their caregivers. You may also write the hours you will be on the unit. Not all nursing programs keep students on the floor for a full shift. After introductions, you are ready for the assessment.

Patient Assessment

The goal of this first morning assessment is to quickly determine the patient's status. Student nurses learn to complete a head-to-toe assessment in the first semester. At first, you will concentrate on normal assessment findings so you can tell what is found in most healthy people. Even if you don't have the correct words for abnormal assessment findings, you are at least beginning to see and hear what is normal and what is not.

Most nurses develop a specific routine or order in the head-to-toe assessment. This helps you cover everything and not miss something. It is helpful to have an assessment form with you as you complete your assessment. Then you can check one system and chart it before you continue to the next. Charting as you go allows you to receive "cues" from the form itself (see Chapter 6 about charting). This helps you remember each thing you are supposed to check.

An experienced nurse can do a quick head-to-toe assessment in about 10 minutes. It will of course take you longer at first. Be sure your patient understands that you will be "checking them out" for about 30 minutes or so. Keeping your patient informed of what you're doing makes them more comfortable.

If your patient wants to close their eyes again after the assessment is done, you can turn out the lights and close the door knowing that you have a good picture of their status. If the patient is awake and ready to begin the day, you can encourage them to sit up in the chair if capable, to be ready for breakfast. Remember the smile, the personal touch and the human contact are all such an important part of each interaction.

Another thing to practice each time you're in the room is *observing* as much as possible. Train yourself when you enter the room to look first at the patient and then at the surroundings: is the patient breathing easily or in distress? Do they converse appropriately and answer questions? When you ask them to turn over, do they do it? What about pain? What intravenous (IV) fluid is hanging? What is the intravenous pump set on? Does this match the orders on the worksheet/ Kardex? Are there any smells you need to pay attention to? Nurses become very astute at observation, but it takes practice. You might as well begin with your first contact.

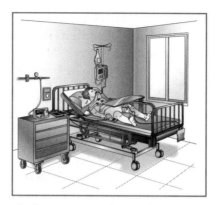

Figure 3-1a   Knocking before opening a door and/or entering a patient's room shows respect.

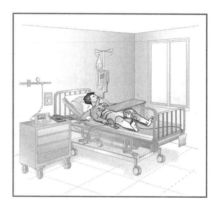

Figure 3-1b   Then as you enter the room, look directly at the patient and walk in with a smile. Next offer a greeting that includes their entire name, for instance "Good morning Mrs. Harrison, my name is Brad and I'll be your student nurse today." Many patients will invite you to call them by their first name; but it is better to use their last name and title until they express a preference. To some cultures or patient age groups using a first name is disrespectful.

As you look at the patient, you actually begin your assessment. What can you tell simply by entering the room and greeting them? General status, for instance whether or not they are: in distress, breathing easily, awake, alert, groggy, slow to respond, able to localize your voice, at ease in their facial features, in a relaxed posture, positioned uncomfortably, etc. Each of these observations helps you recognize what the patient might need and thus begins your assessment.

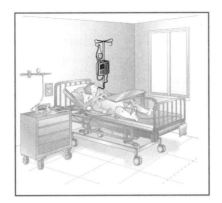

Figure 3-1c   Once you are assured about your patient's general status, check the IV. The fluid that is hanging and the rate showing on the pump should match the physician's order. The site (where the IV actually enters the patient's skin) should not show any redness, swelling, tenderness, or drainage.

If there are other pieces of equipment, check each of them. . .suction should be set to the proper level. . .oxygen rate and delivery method needs to match the orders. . .tube feedings are controlled by a pump and again, specific orders for type of feeding and rate need to be correct. . .any telemetry leads need to be properly positioned and in good contact with the skin.

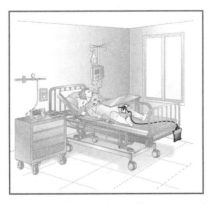

Figure 3-1d   The foley catheter bag collects urine. Notice the color (it should be light yellow colored), the quantity in the bag and the tubing. The urine only drains by gravity; there is never suction applied to the catheter. So all tubing needs to flow downhill. If parts of the tubing hang low, in such a way that the urine would have to travel uphill to get into the collection bag, the urine may back up into the bladder and could cause infection. To protect against this, each catheter has a small clip to hold it up on the sheets. The catheter tube also needs to be anchored, either with tape or a soft Velcro holder to assure it doesn't pull.

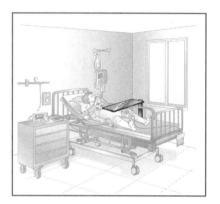

Figure 3-1e   Hospital rooms have a table that telescopes up and down to different heights and can be positioned over the hospital bed. Check that it is clean (you may find urinals, old food, used tissues, etc.). A cluttered, dirty over-bed table can become a place for germs to grow and also can discourage the patient from wanting to eat. Necessary items should be within reach: tissues, water, phone, etc.

Then you will accomplish the purpose of entering the room. When you are ready to leave, again make it a habit to check specific things before you go.

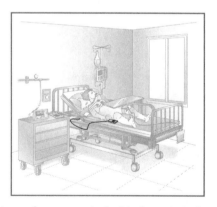

Figure 3-1f   For patient safety assure the bed is down in its lowest position.

The nurse call light and bed controls should be within reach.

The pathway to the bathroom needs to be clear; make sure no equipment or patient belongings are in the way.

Check the Orders

After assessment, it is time to head for a quick chart check, not to read the chart but to look for medication orders. Specifically, you need to check orders and compare to the medication record (usually called the medication administration record, or MAR). When nurses give medications, we work from the MAR. It is very important that the doctor's order was transcribed properly onto the MAR. So after assessment, check the MAR to assure it is correct. (At first, you may only have time to check for the morning medications at this point in the day; check later medications later when you have more time.)

Have your primary nurse help you be sure that each of your morning medications is actually on the unit and that you haven't missed any. Sometimes medications are in a box with the patient's name on it, sometimes in a machine that dispenses them from a little drawer or other times in a medication refrigerator. The primary nurse will help you know where to look. If the medications are not there, call the pharmacy to get them. All of this preparation work before giving medications takes time and is the reason you don't wait until the ordered time before getting ready.

You will likely need to look up some of the drugs. Although you will have a pharmacology class, there is no way nurses can memorize all the drugs we give! You will be using your personal digital assistant, the hospital intranet or a drug reference book to check for drug information for the rest of your career. The purpose of looking them up is for a quick review, not a long study session. Marking the page(s) allows quick reference later. Some students prepare index cards of the drugs they give for future reference and to help memorize the common drugs. Look them up, take notes as needed and check any laboratory tests (labs) or vital signs you are directed to know before you give the drug.

For instance, many patients are given a diuretic drug to get rid of fluid. When the body urinates out the extra fluid, some electrolytes may be lost. Potassium is a common electrolyte that can get low when patients are on certain diuretics. The drug book will tell you to check the labs before giving the diuretic or the potassium replacement. Makes sense, huh? Practical nursing implications like this will be written for most of the drugs you will give.

Having this information in mind and assuring the drug is actually on the unit before your instructor comes to give morning medications with you really makes you a star! It also makes you safer for your patient care. Don't you love it when everyone wins?! And notice that all of this has happened in the first hour and a half of your shift. You have already met your primary nurse, taken report, assessed your patient and looked up and prepared your morning medications. Phew! Good work. You are taking charge of the shift when you begin like this.

Giving Medications with Your Instructor

Since you have assessed your patient, checked the MAR against the doctor's orders, looked up drug information and assured that the ordered medications are on the unit, you are now ready to give the medications with your instructor. Once you have demonstrated that you follow proper procedures, your instructor will likely let you give your medications under the supervision of your primary nurse. At first, though, you will only give medications with your instructor present.

Hospitals have standardized times for most medication administration. Nine o'clock in the morning is common for the first daily drugs to be given, with a window of an hour before or after the ordered time being considered "on time." In some institutions, the window for on-time administration is shorter, so check with your instructor. When your instructor joins you at the medication cart or in the medication room, systematically go through the MAR and show him or her what you are going to give.

Explain what each drug is for and what labs or physical findings you checked. Answer any questions the instructor has. Then the two of you will go to the patient's room to give the drugs. In nursing fundamentals, you will learn that there are at least five rights of medication administration. You will demonstrate them in front of the instructor: right patient, right drug, right dose, right route, and right time. Some programs add a sixth: right documentation after you have given the drug; other sources are beginning to expand the "rights" to include right to refuse, etc.

The key to success in medication administration is to be prepared. By the time you finish morning medications, it will likely be about 9:30 or 10:30 and you will

---

BOX 3-1   Preparation of Medications Before the Instructor Arrives

- Assure the MAR is transcribed properly from the doctor's orders
- Look up the drugs as needed
- Assure the drug is on the unit
- Assure you can state for each drug:
  - What benefit will this drug have for the patient?
  - Are there any physical signs to check before giving this (i.e., blood pressure, pulse, etc.)?
  - Are there any labs to know before giving this (i.e., electrolytes, etc.)?
  - Calculate any dosage as needed
  - How will you evaluate if the drug is effective?
  - Is the patient allergic to this drug or a drug in its class?
- Have all needed equipment ready, including water for the patient to drink
- Be sure the patient has a wrist band on for identification and an allergy bracelet

need a break! It is good to get in the habit of taking a quick break, getting a drink and using the restroom. Some nurses work through an entire shift without stopping. That practice leads to fatigue and burnout (not to mention bladder infections!) and is not good practice. There is usually a staff break room with a bathroom and a place to sit down for a few minutes right on the unit.

Continuing the Morning

When you return from your break, check in with your primary nurse and check your patient(s). You can help them at this time with their morning care, complete the assessment if there were parts you deferred, chart what has been completed, plan with the patient their preferences for the rest of the shift, etc. Spending time in the patient's room early in the shift increases your familiarity and comfort with them and builds their trust.

While you are performing these activities with and for them, ask questions and get them talking. It is a great opportunity to find out what brought them to the hospital and what the doctor has told them so far. Most people appreciate talking about themselves, and will share quite a bit of information if you invite it. Listening also demonstrates the human side that is such an integral part of nursing care. It will probably be about 10:00 or 10:30 when you finish this part of your shift.

Reading the Chart

Now is a good time to read through the patient's chart before you go to lunch. Of course, you won't read every word of every page. Most hospital charts are at the nurses' station filed by room number. They flip open at the top and have dividers for each important section. Find out where you can sit as you read the chart; most hospitals do not want the charts far from the nurses' station because all caregivers use them.

As more charting is completed on the computer, much of what we used to read from the paper chart will be found on the computer. Your instructor and your primary nurse will help you know where to find the chart and reports you need. Here is a suggested order for quickly gathering what you need from a chart, whether in hard copy or electronic chart:

BOX 3-2   Reading a Patient's Chart

1. Begin with the doctor's H&P
2. Find the nurse's admission assessment and read it
3. Check the most recent physician's progress note(s)
4. If surgery was performed, read the operation report; if there are important diagnostic tests, read the reports of their findings
5. Read any other pertinent consults or reports

Let's look at each of these parts separately.

1. **Begin with the doctor's history and physical (H&P).**
   This is the best place to start because it summarizes the patient's medical history and describes exactly what brought them to the hospital (this is called the chief complaint [cc]). The H&P is a typed report, so it is easy to read. There will likely be words you haven't learned yet; it's helpful to make a list of these and look them up or ask their meaning as you go through the shift. Sometimes, you will not find the H&P on the chart. This is usually because the patient was admitted during the previous night and the H&P has not been transcribed yet.

2. **Find the nurse's admission assessment and read it.**
   Some of the information on the nurse's admission assessment will be the same as what you read on the H&P. However, nurses ask about other things, and you will get a more complete picture of your patient. Reading the admission note will also help you learn what to ask when you admit a patient.

3. **Check the most recent physician's progress notes.**
   Each day, the doctor visits the patient in the hospital and writes a note called a "progress note." These progress notes are very important because they literally tell you what the physician is thinking. Unfortunately, in most facilities they are handwritten and are often difficult to read. (Have you heard jokes about doctor's poor handwriting? They are often true!!). There is a format that most doctors follow when they write their progress notes.

   The note usually begins with a narrative comment about the current status. Some physicians separate out the comments the patient makes directly about their feelings from the observations the physician makes themselves. Patient comments are considered subjective information (labeled S, if the physician uses that format) and the doctor's observations are labeled O, for objective data. The first comment may be something like this:

   S—"My incision hurts."

   O—slight redness, no drainage, good skin approximation

   If the note does not separate out subjective and objective information, the physician may simply begin the note with the entry, "Incision clear, no drainage and good approximation, slight redness. Pt c/o (complains of) pain at incision." Get the idea?

   Next, the physician's note will summarize the assessment findings. This is often labeled with PE (for physical exam). Under the PE, it is usual to include abbreviations for body systems. The assessment usually begins with pertinent vitals (short for vital signs which include blood pressure, pulse, respirations and temperature), then goes to HEENT (meaning head, eyes, ears, nose and throat), NECK, CHEST, ABD (meaning abdomen), NEURO (meaning neurologic),

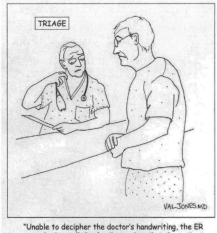

"Unable to decipher the doctor's handwriting, the ER nurse had to tell the family member that the patient was either 'released' or 'deceased.'"

EXTR (extremities) and LABS (referring to laboratory test results and sometimes diagnostics). Here is an example of what the physical exam section of the note might look like, omitting the LABS section, which is discussed next:

Vitals: 136/65, 88, 18, T 38 C

HEENT: unremarkable

NECK: unremarkable

CHEST: fine crackles bilaterally at bases

ABD: soft, slight swelling. Midline abdominal incision with staples intact. Minor guarding on palpation. BS active

NEURO: CN I–XII intact, sensory, cerebellar and motor exams WNLs, DTRs 2+ and bilat = Patient is A&O with intact short term memory

EXTR: no cyanosis or edema

Of course it would not be typed for easy reading and you would need to ask about certain abbreviations and medical terms you may not know yet, but this gives you the general outline similar to what most physicians use.

If you read this note out loud, you would say "blood pressure is 136/65, pulse 88, respirations 18 per minute and the temperature is 38°C (or 100.6°F). Assessment of the head, eyes, ears, nose, throat and neck are normal. Listening to the chest with a stethoscope, there is slight sound of fluid in the bases of the lungs on both sides. The abdomen is soft and has slight swelling. There is an incision running vertically down the middle of the belly, and the staples are holding it together. Listening to the belly with a stethoscope, there are active gurgling bowel sounds heard. Cranial nerves I through XII are working fine and other neurologic checks are within normal limits. Deep tendon reflexes are moderately strong and equal on both sides. The patient is alert and knows who she is, where she is, and what day it is and remembers specifics about this morning. Neither the arms nor the legs have any purple or blue discoloration, nor do they have fluid retention." See why the terminology and abbreviations are used? They convey more while requiring less writing.

Laboratory results are often reported by physicians in their Progress Notes in a strange looking shorthand shape with numbers in it. The shape and its corresponding labs look like this:

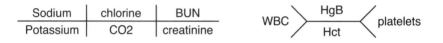

These figures would be drawn in the Progress Note, with the actual numbers in the spaces for each of the lab results on that patient. This demonstrates that the physician looked up the labs and considered them in the Progress Note report. In class, you will learn what these abbreviations mean, the normal ranges for labs (most labs will include normal ranges on the report of results) and the significance of abnormal findings for each condition or disease process.

After the physician has recorded the PE findings, the next section will usually be what conclusions are drawn. Often, this is recorded after the PE section as "Imp" (meaning impression). Impression can also be translated into diagnosis. It is here that you will discover what the doctor thinks is going on with the patient now based on the latest diagnostics, patient presentation, labs, etc. In other words, sometimes when a patient is first admitted, the diagnosis is not yet known for sure. Once results are back from labs and tests, the doctor will figure out the actual diagnosis and write it under "Imp". Thus the first "admitting diagnosis" won't be changed, but the updated, actual diagnosis and/or other patient problems are now identified and listed. It is critical that nurses are aware of this update!

After the impressions are given, the final part of the note is the Plan (often abbreviated simply with a P). Lists of orders, medication changes, consults to be obtained, etc., follow. You can see why this section is so important to read!

After you have completed the Progress Note, check for surgery notes.

4. **If surgery was performed, read the operation report; if there are important diagnostic tests, read the reports of their findings.**

Findings of diagnostic tests and procedures will have summaries typed. These are easy to read and critical for understanding your patient's status. Again, you are likely to read medical terminology that you aren't familiar with, so take notes and ask questions. The more you read, the more quickly you will build up the terms in your own vocabulary.

5. **Read any other pertinent consults or reports.**

    It is not unusual for the physician who admitted the patient to call other specialist doctors in on the case to help with either diagnosis or treatment. These doctors are referred to as "consultants." After they have seen the patient, they will dictate and/or write a consult note. Sometimes, it is done in the body of the Progress Notes section. Other times, it is given a separate section titled "Consults." Reading through these reports allows you to know what is found for that particular patient symptom or system and also lets you learn what types of problems each medical specialty addresses.

    The time it takes to complete a chart review will vary quite a bit as some charts are thin and some are very thick with pages of information.

Hopefully, you will complete the chart review by lunch time. Before you leave for lunch, go back into your patient's room and see if they need anything. Make a charting entry at this time. Charting as you go through the shift is another good habit to cultivate from the beginning (see Chapter 6).

Find your primary nurse and give a quick report before going to lunch. Any time you leave the unit, let your nurse know so the patient(s) will be covered while you're gone. Some instructors have their clinical students eat lunch together as a way of building a sense of cohesiveness and support. If you are working a 12-hour shift, some instructors hold "postconference" in the middle of the shift to break up the long hours and to address any questions or problems the students may have.

When you return to the floor after lunch, make rounds again on your patient(s). Help them with anything they need, chart, and listen to them. This is a nice time to get to know them better. You may have more medicines to give at this time, so prepare as you did for morning medications and give them with your instructor.

In the afternoons, you can more easily plan for patient teaching, walking with your patients, etc. Take advantage of going with them to any tests or procedures if you are allowed. This is a great way to learn about other departments and see what your patient experiences as they have different tests.

Another hint during the shift: go in the patient's room when you see other caregivers enter. If the doctor visits, being there allows you to hear what the patient is told, help the patient to ask any questions they may have had but are too hesitant to ask, and be clear on what is planned. Some physicians encourage students to ask questions during these physician rounds. Likewise, your presence during visits by therapists provides a great opportunity to learn what other caregivers do for our patients in general and for your individual patient so you can follow up.

If you have been working an 8-hour shift, your time is almost done. You may have more medication to give, treatments to complete or skills to do. Hopefully, your instructor has checked in with you a couple of times to answer questions, see your progress and supervise as you do procedures or skills. See Chapter 7 for suggestions about working with your instructor. At the end of the shift, you will usually attend postconference. This is covered in Chapter 9. The following tables take the discussion covered in this chapter and put it in an easy reference form as a suggested timeline for managing a shift. Of course, any "plan" is subject to change as patient needs and learning opportunities present themselves.

Phew! A nurse's workday is packed and busy; but if you approach it with a plan in mind, you can complete what you need to by the end of the shift. Let's put all that we have talked about into a timetable chart for your reference.

TABLE 3-1   Time Management Chart

Time Management—8-hour shift
Student Nurse Planning

This timetable is a suggestion of how to plan your clinical day. The better organized you are, the safer care you will give and the more controlled your day will be. Of course, adjust as needed.

Time	Action	Rationale
0630	Preconference; meet primary nurse; choose patient(s); plan day	Clarity in focus and plan assists in safe care
0700	Take report; complete student worksheet according to Kardex	Communication between shifts aids in patient care; worksheet assists time management
0730	Patient rounds; quick assessment; document as you go to assure accuracy and time management	Assures student familiarity with assigned patients; assists in prioritizing and patient input to day's care
0800	Check MAR with doctor orders in chart; check medication box for 0900 medications	Assure accuracy of transcription; assure medications on floor when needed
0830	Look up any medication info, lab info or recheck any assessment info needed for med administration; provide a.m. care	Allows factual basis for nursing care and safety in medication administration
0900	Give 0900 medications with instructor	Hospital policy allows 60 minutes either side of scheduled time as "on time" medication administration
1000	Make rounds; coordinate with primary nurse regarding patient status; complete more thorough assessment if needed; assure charting is up to date	Frequent patient contact assures student is current; coordination between caregivers meets patient needs best; charting as you work increases accuracy of charting and keeps student on time
	Use restroom	Minimize risk of student urinary tract infection

TABLE 3-1   Time Management Chart

Time	Action	Rationale
1030	Complete morning care and patient treatments; check chart for pertinent medical history, consult reports, etc.	Assures complete care and understanding of patient condition
	Give report to instructor	Allows practice at proper professional report style; gives instructor opportunity to share info and give feedback about patient condition/nursing care
1100	Take lunch break; students are responsible for signing off to primary nurse and patient before leaving floor	Improves student health; allows mental and physical break so students can give optimal care; communication essential for patient safety
1130	Return to floor; make rounds on patient(s) with care and teaching as indicated; update charting	Assure current patient status; provides for patient needs
1200	Pass lunch trays; assist with care; update documentation; check 1300 medications	Provides needed care; prepares for timely medication administration
1230	Give 1300 medications with instructor; check with patient for any last needs before leaving floor; report off to primary before leaving floor; assure documentation complete	Provides timely safe medication administration; communication essential for safe care
1300	Leave for postconference; use restroom; get a drink	Avoid student health problems
1315	Postconference	Share information; discuss problems; update plans and skills
	Thanks for working hard!	

Time Management—12-hour shift
Student Nurse Planning

This timetable is a suggestion of how to plan your clinical day. The better organized you are, the safer care you will give and the more controlled your day will be. Of course, adjust as needed and as your instructor advises.

Time	Action	Rationale
0630	Preconference; get assigned primary nurse; plan day	Clarity in focus and plan assists in safe care
0700	Take report; complete student worksheet according to Kardex	Communication between shifts aids in patient care; worksheet assists time management

(continues)

TABLE 3-1   Time Management Chart *(Continued)*

Time	*Action*	*Rationale*
0730	Patient rounds; quick assessment; document as you go to assure accuracy and time management	Assures student familiarity with assigned patients; assists in prioritizing and patient input to day's care
0800	Check MAR with doctor orders in chart; check med box for 0900 medications; care nurse assist patients up and pass trays	Assure accuracy of transcription; assure medications on floor when needed
0830	Look up any medication info, lab info or recheck any assessment info needed for med administration; care nurse provide a.m. care	Allows factual basis for nursing care and med administration
0900	Give 0900 medications with instructor	Hospital policy allows 30 minutes either side of scheduled time as "on time" medication administration
1000	Make rounds; coordinate with primary nurse regarding patient status; complete more thorough assessment if needed; assure charting is up to date	Frequent patient contact assures student is current; coordination between caregivers meets patient needs best
	Use restroom	Minimize risk of student urinary tract infection
1030	Complete morning care and patient treatments; check chart for pertinent medical history, consult reports, etc. Give report to instructor	Assures complete care and understanding of patient condition; allows practice at proper professional report style; gives instructor opportunity to share info and give feedback about patient condition/ nursing care.
1100	Lunch break; students responsible for signing off to primary nurse and patient before leaving floor	Improves student health; allows mental and physical break so students can give optimal care; communication essential for patient safety.
	Student lunch/conference with instructor; bring lunch to conference room; bring worksheet	Collaboration with faculty improves quality of clinical day, assists students to begin required paperwork; after the first 3 weeks, this lunch conference may be abandoned if not needed
1230	Return to floor; check in with primary nurse; make rounds on patient(s); update assessments and charting; check 1300 medications	Assure current patient status; assure continuity of care

TABLE 3-1   Time Management Chart

Time	Action	Rationale
1300	Give 1300 medications with instructor or with primary nurse if approved	Provides timely safe medication administration; communication essential for safe care.
1330	Assure charting is up-to-date; continue patient care and teaching	Efficiency is enhanced if charting is completed as you go
1400	Check for any new orders on patients; provide cares, treatments, etc.; tally totals of intake and output (I&O)	Assure compliance with medical orders; efficiency of work
1430	Prepare for report with instructor and primary nurse; at beginning of semester, listen to report as primary gives it—later, student will give report to oncoming shift	Communication important for continuity of care
1500	Give report to oncoming evening shift, whether nurse or student	Some facilities no longer have 3–11 shift; instead, all are 12-hour shifts: 7 a.m.–7 p.m. and 7 p.m.–7 a.m.
1530	Patient rounds, assessment and charting	Meets standards of care for assessment
1600	Patient teaching; chart review for background information, consult reports, etc.	
1730	Check with patient(s) for any last needs before leaving floor; report off to primary before leaving floor; assure documentation complete	Communication is key to meeting patient needs
1800	Postconference	Thank you for working hard

Worksheets

Nursing is a demanding profession. Many tasks are required of the nurse during the shift, and it helps to have a worksheet when starting out. This will cue you of tasks due and assure that you have completed all of your responsibilities by the end of your shift. A worksheet also provides information you can refer to during the shift without pulling the chart again and helps you give report when shift is done. You can fold it and keep it in your pocket or on a clipboard at the workstation or medication cart.

A worksheet will not be used in a nursing home, intensive care unit or during observation or community experiences. When you are in these and other special areas, you will likely have only one patient, and it is easier to track what is required. For instance, the charting in an intensive care unit becomes the cue for each nursing task. But when you are working on a medical or surgical (med-surg) unit keeping track of two or more patients, a worksheet is invaluable.

There are many different formats you can use for a nursing worksheet. Each has a place for demographics about your patient, orders that need to be followed and any other information that helps you stay on target. Some facilities have preprinted worksheets for the nurses, some nurses have developed their own style and format and some nurses do not use any worksheet. Facilities where charting is done on computer often receive a computer printout page(s) for each patient that can be converted into a worksheet.

Try different formats, ask other nurses, check with your instructor and see what works for you, but most student nurses find it very helpful to have something to help remind them of all that needs to be done.

The *most important piece of advice about a worksheet* is to build in a system for seeing at a glance what time things are due and if they have been done and charted. Using circled numbers representing the time a task is due really helps. Then when the task is done, you slash a diagonal line through the time. When the task is done AND charted, you slash a diagonal line in the other direction and "X" out the task!

Let's say you had to give medications for this patient at 0900, 1100 and 1300. Under the column of your worksheet for Medication (see examples at the end of this chapter), write 9, 11 and 13 and circle each number ⑨⑪⑬. After you have *given* all of the 9 o'clock medications, you will slash diagonally in one direction to indicate the task is done. So it would look like this ⑨, meaning you gave the 9 o'clock medications. After you had charted that you gave the medication, slash it out on your worksheet diagonally the other direction like this ⑨. Now, in one glance at your worksheet, you can see that you both gave *and* charted the 9 o'clock medications. Hooray!

Setting your worksheet up with circled times that can be crossed out is really a helpful organizing tool. Some of the things that have times associated with them include giving medications, helping a patient turn and change position every 2 hours, reminding a patient to breathe deeply and cough, assisting with an Incentive Spirometer (a piece of equipment the patient uses to inhale deeply), totaling up intake and output, checking the blood sugar by pricking the finger (called glucometer check), walking with a patient (called ambulating), changing a dressing and as many other things as you can think of.

See how valuable a worksheet is in keeping you organized at a glance? Another benefit is that you have basic orders at your fingertips so you don't have to run to the chart to look things up constantly. For instance, the first section includes the patient's name, age, medical record number, doctor's name, allergies and code status (code status speaks to whether we resuscitate the patient if their heart stops: full code if they want resuscitation, no code if they do not want heroic intervention).

Other sections will have diet, activity and intravenous fluid orders (type of fluid and rate). Preparing all of this on your worksheet or printing it from the computer is very handy when you need to know something quickly. Since you carry the worksheet but not the entire chart, this gives you much of what you need to know.

Nurses who use a worksheet also benefit from taking report notes on the back of the worksheet during change of shift report. That gives them a quick reference to the patient's status from the previous shift. See the end of the chapter for some sample worksheets. It takes some practice to discover what format works for you. Have fun with it!

Nursing Care Versus Task Completion

Just because the worksheet tracks task completion doesn't mean that nursing is simply crossing jobs/tasks/orders off of a worksheet. Completing the responsibilities of the job is important and does help your patient. However, completing those tasks while you are actually *thinking* about what is going on is best! While you help someone complete a task or goal, notice what you can about it and what it tells you about the patient's condition.

For instance, nurses spend time helping patients walk. Ambulation (walking) is beneficial for circulation, muscles, breathing, emotions and increasing intestinal peristalsis. So encouraging people to walk and helping them ambulate safely is vital to the patient progressing. But while walking with the patient, a good nurse will notice other aspects in addition to the simple act of walking (or whatever other task is being completed). What else do we want to know? How does the patient feel? Is he or she steady? Does pain worsen or improve with the action? What is the breathing pattern like? What happens to the heart rate with activity? Does the patient's color change with activity?

During morning care, while helping people get cleaned up and dressed, the nurse can make note of the patient's degree of physical ability (or inability). It is a perfect time to engage them in conversation about how much they understand about their disease process: what have they been told? What does it mean to them? What kind of options does the doctor discuss? Were they told the problem can be totally solved or will there be ongoing problems? How does the patient expect this to impact their lives?

Task completion time is also a perfect opportunity to listen to the patient and learn more about their history, goals, expectations, family, supports, etc. Ask questions that get them talking. The more we learn about our patients, the more compassion we show as our understanding of them as human beings increases and the more interesting our job is, too. The nurse who cares benefits both herself and her patient. On your worksheet, you will be crossing off tasks, but in the nurse's notes you will add narratives about the story that is unfolding regarding the patient's situation.

We are also observing for the effects of medications that we have given or treatments that have been completed while we go about other aspects of our job. For instance, we may have given a drug to decrease nausea. It is important to ask if the drug has decreased the nausea. The same is true for drugs for pain, for decreasing blood pressure, or getting rid of a headache, etc. See the pattern? During the task completion, we have an opportunity to follow up how other interventions have affected our patients.

Some worksheet examples follow. The first worksheet is the form that can be used for one or two patients.

Worksheet 3-A   Student Nurse Worksheet

Student _____   Date _____   Primary nurse _____   Floor _____

Place patient sticker here: room number, name, age, sex, admission date, admitting diagnosis, physician	Assessment	Activity	Diet	Vital signs	IV and I&O	Labs and tests	Medications
					Site / Fluid / Rate / Credit / Intake / Output / Drsng change / Tubing change		
Allergies Code status							
					Site / Fluid / Rate / Credit / Intake / Output / Drsng change / Tubing change		
Allergies Code status							

Worksheet 3-A Author's Notes

At the beginning of the shift, take information and orders from the computer print-out of your patient or from the Kardex, depending on what your facility uses, and put the information on the worksheet with time cues circled to keep you on target through the shift. The worksheet can be folded and carried in your pocket or put on a clipboard for easy reference during the shift. Cross out the tasks as you complete and chart them.

Create a worksheet whenever you are working on a hospital unit. Worksheets do not help much in a nursing home or in an intensive care unit. You won't need a worksheet when you are working in an observation unit either (see Chapter 8). However, on the medical or surgical unit they are invaluable. Another note: the basic worksheet can be adapted for special areas like postpartum. In those areas, you would add aspects that are common to all patients there, but not used on other floors, like para and gravida status, episiotomy, baby's weight and APGAR, etc.

HIPAA—a note about privacy: nurses hear quite a bit of information that is private and sensitive. Our patients have a right to expect us to keep that personal information confidential. The very fact that a specific person is in the hospital is part of the protected information. Nurses and students cultivate in themselves a practice of protecting privacy: we don't talk about our patients by their names when in public places (for instance, in the cafeteria with fellow students), we close computer screens when we leave the computer and when we have print material that has personal information (like our worksheet), we cover it with a piece of blank paper so no one passing our clipboard can see names and information.

Worksheet 3-B   Student Nurse Worksheet

Student _your name here_   Date _current date_   Primary nurse _write the name of your primary nurse_ (the nurse who works on the floor, and who is assigned the patient you have)   Floor you are working on _the floor_

Place patient sticker here: room number, name, age, sex, admission date, admitting diagnosis, physician	Assessment	Activity	Diet	Vital signs	IV and I&O	Labs and tests	Medications
Room 312 Gloria Smith, 85 year old, F MR# 54321 Admitted 02/03 Pneumonia and sepsis Dr. Jones Allergies Penicillin Code status DNR	⑧	BR ⑦ ⑨ ⑪ ⑬	PEG tube cont. @ 65 irrigate 50 cc water each shift ⑬	⑧ ⑫	Site L wrist Fluid Rate 5L Credit Intake Output Foley Drsng change peg drsng ⑬		⑨ ⑪
Allergies Code status					Site Fluid Rate Credit Intake Output Drsng change Tubing change		

Worksheet 3-B   Author's Notes

This is an example of a worksheet that has been prepared by the beginning student nurse for her patient (one patient).

First column: Demographics. Some facilities use preprinted stickers which have all of this information on them; you peel one off and affix it to the worksheet. You can also print the information on the page. MR = medical record number. Code status refers to whether the patient wants to be resuscitated if their heart and breathing stop. DNR = do not resuscitate. When this lady dies, she does not want CPR performed or drugs and defibrillation used to "save" her. If the patient has no restrictions and wants everything used, they are termed a "full code" status. Nurses need to know each patient's preference so we can respond appropriately.

Second column: Assessment. This reminds you to complete a morning assessment and allows a space to jot any pertinent findings.

Third column: Activity. This lady cannot get out of bed, BR = bed rest. So the student cued herself to move the patient from side to side every 2 hours to prevent complications of immobility, not by writing "turn every 2 hours," but by putting circled times on the page.

Fourth column: Diet. Physicians will specify diet orders. This lady has a tube into her stomach and the nurses hang liquid formula in a bag controlled by a pump to deliver nutrition constantly. The order = 65 cc/hour, plus irrigating with 50 cc water every shift. The student cued herself to do this at 1300.

Fifth column: Vital signs (VS). This term refers to blood pressure, pulse, respiration and temperature. The student found orders to take VS every 4 hours. Instead of writing "every 4 hours" in the column, write the times and circle them, then you are cued to remember.

Sixth column: IV/I&O. The worksheet shows there is a SL (saline lock) in the left wrist. SL = IV access but closed off, without fluids running all the time. This gives a place for intermittent IV drugs to be connected when needed. At the end of the shift, it is common to add up all of the fluids that the patient took in and everything that was excreted. Noted on this worksheet is that the patient has a Foley, which is a catheter in her bladder to catch the urine.

Seventh column: Labs and tests. On this worksheet, nothing is needed for this patient. Sometimes, orders will include things that go in this column (i.e., what test results are being awaited, or cue to prick the finger for blood sugar [glucometer test] as we do for diabetics).

Eighth column: Medications. The student checked the MAR and wrote the times that medications are scheduled.

Worksheet 3-C   Student Nurse Worksheet

Student _your name here_   Date _current date_   Primary nurse _write the name of your primary nurse (the nurse who works on the floor, who is assigned the patient you have)_   Floor _you are working on the floor_

Place patient sticker here: room number, name, age, sex, admission date, admitting diagnosis, physician	Assessment	Activity	Diet	Vital signs	IV and I&O	Labs and tests	Medications
Room 312 Gloria Smith, 85 year old, F MR# 54321 Admitted 02/03 Pneumonia and sepsis Dr. Jones Allergies Penicillin Code status DNR	⊗ Can not state name or follow commands Diminished breath sounds	BR ⊗R ⊗L ⑪ ⑬	PEG tube cont. @ 65 irrigate 50 cc water each shift ⑬	⊗ 112/73, 92, 24, T 37.5C (99.6°F) ⑫	Site L wrist Fluid Rate SL Credit Intake Output Foley Drsng change peg drsng ⑬	wbc count is down	⊗ ⑪
					Site Fluid Rate Credit Intake Output Drsng change Tubing change		
Allergies Code status							

Worksheet 3-C Author's Notes

This is the same worksheet but later in the shift, about 1100 before the student goes to lunch.

You can see at a glance that the student has completed the assessment and charted it. You can also see what some of the important findings were. The student did not write the entire assessment here. That would waste time as the full assessment needs to be charted in the permanent chart. The student's worksheet is not a part of the medical record; you are using it to remember things to do and things to report.

Under activity, BR means the patient is on bed rest. The patient's position was changed at 7 o'clock and 9 o'clock. At 7, the patient was positioned on her right side, and at 9 moved over to the left side. See how easy it is?!

The VS column shows what the morning findings were. Because there is only one slash mark on the 8 o'clock VS, we know that the VS were taken but not yet charted. It is best to chart right away so everyone caring for the patient can see what the current VS are, but at least with a glance at the worksheet, you can see what isn't done yet.

Although there was not a cued time in the Labs column, you can see that some lab results have been returned. Specifically, the student notes that the white blood cell (WBC) count is down. This is important because it is one of the ways the body fights an infection (remember the patient's diagnosis is pneumonia? That is an infection of the lungs). A healthy person's wbc will go up as the body fights an infection. An older person sometimes cannot create enough wbcs to fight infections; or the wbc may have been up earlier and is now coming down because antibiotics are helping to fight the infection. See how there is much to think about, not simply a lab finding to write down? It is fun to understand what the findings may indicate. Discuss this kind of thing with your primary nurse and instructor.

And lastly, we can see that the morning medications have been given and charted.

The student can look at the worksheet before leaving for lunch and may decide to complete the 11 o'clock tasks before leaving the floor.

Looks like the student is on track with to a shift that is under control!

Worksheet 3-D   Student Nurse Worksheet

Student _your name here_   Date _current date_   Primary nurse _write the name of your primary nurse (the nurse who works on the floor, who is assigned the patient you have)_   Floor _you are working on the floor_

Place patient sticker here: room number, name, age, sex, admission date, admitting diagnosis, physician	Assessment	Activity	Diet	Vital signs	IV and I&O	Labs and tests	Medications
Room 312	⊗	BR	PEG tube cont. @ 65	⊗ 112/73, 92, 24, T 37.5C (99.6°F)	Site L wrist Fluid Rate SL Credit	wbc count is down	⊗
Gloria Smith, 85 year old, F MR# 54321 Admitted 02/03 Pneumonia and sepsis	Can not state name or follow commands	⊗⊗R ⊗L	irrigate 50 cc water each shift ⑬	⊗	Intake Output Foley		⊗
Dr. Jones	Diminished breath sounds	⊗B ⊗ R		110/72, 96, 22 T 37C	Drsng change peg dressing ⑬		
Allergies Penicillin Code status DNR							
			Site Fluid Rate Credit			
				Intake Output		
Allergies Code status					Drsng change Tubing change		

Worksheet 3-D Author's Notes

Now it is almost time to leave the floor and go to postconference (see Chapter 9).

Checking the worksheet at this point shows what needs to be finished before leaving the floor. The student needs to irrigate the PEG tube and change the dressing around it, chart those final things and then can leave the floor knowing that all of the responsibilities were met.

Hooray!

A couple of extra notes about the worksheet:

- If you planned to do something and then could not complete it because of changes, instead of crossing out with diagonal lines, you can simply cross off the time cue with a note why the task wasn't completed. For instance: if *1300* medication administration was not given because a medication for blood pressure was ordered, but the blood pressure was too low and so the student, after discussion with the primary nurse, decided not to give the med. You can indicate that in this manner: *13* and then write *"held BP 96/55."*

- We are often asked to get something for our patients or their family members. When you agree to bring something or ask about something, be sure you don't forget! Your patient is counting on you and if you don't follow up, or you are late in your promise, trust is lost. So, the worksheet can become a way to assure you actually follow through. Let's say that your patient asked for an extra blanket, since it was cold last night. You agree to bring a blanket, but plan to do it after lunch. Put it in a time circle like other tasks *1230 blanket*. After lunch, when you check your worksheet again, you will remember your promise and get the blanket and cross it off. Other aspects of our human relationship with our patient, compassion and respect, has been demonstrated!

- Another cue nurses need is to follow up after giving what is called a "p.r.n." medication. There are times when a patient experiences some uncomfortable feeling, and the nurse gives a one-time "as needed" (that's what p.r.n. means) medication. Professionalism requires that we follow up after giving it to be sure that it helped. You might give extra p.r.n. medications for pain, nausea or headache, etc. Because it wasn't scheduled, you need to add it to the worksheet, and add a follow-up time. Let's say the patient asked for pain medicine at 0945, so you gave a pill. It takes pills about 45–60 minutes to work, so we would want to check back with the patient about 1045. It might look like this: *0945 pain med 1045 follow up*. Then you would cross off the follow up 1045 time after you had done that.

Chapter 4
Seeing Your Patient's Big Picture

The patient in the bed doesn't feel good. Their hair is not done nicely. They are dressed in a hospital gown that is less than flattering and at times embarrassingly revealing. They are feeling vulnerable and threatened and, sometimes, that does not bring out the best aspects of a person's personality. From the student nurse's perspective, it helps to remember that, in their own "normal" world, these people—our patients—are functional human beings. They have jobs or are retired. They have people who love them and depend on them. Of course, we know that, but it helps if we require ourselves as caregivers to consider it consciously and try to understand.

Your clinical experience as a student will involve you going into the hospital for a shift or two each week. Time spent in clinical care of real patients, as discussed in the previous chapters, allows you the opportunity to provide compassionate care to people in need, to practice time management skills and to take what you have learned in the classroom and apply it to actual patients. There is a challenge in this scenario, though: you are with them for only a slice of time.

In this one snippet of time, this one shift each week, the student needs to make a concerted effort to get a big picture of this person. What roles does he or she usually play? What responsibilities does he or she have? Just who are these people we call our patients? And how does this one shift we are involved in fit into the whole hospital scene? Our one shift is not going to be their entire hospital stay. The student nurse needs to try to understand this part of the picture, too.

This chapter presents an exercise to assist the student nurse to meet this challenge: **Where were they? Where are they? Where are they going?**

You already possess the two skills needed to master this exercise: (1) compassion about people and (2) ability to listen. Isn't it reassuring that this important aspect is one that is so easy?! Not only is it easy, but approaching your patients with a plan to understand their "big picture" also cultivates the holistic human aspect that underlies all of nursing. After years of experience, you will likely accomplish this exercise mentally all throughout your shift. But for now, make a habit of cultivating it actively and consciously. Ask yourself those three questions to get the whole picture. Let's discuss the three questions, and how to use them to gain the big picture.

Where Were They?

Begin by discovering your patient's past, not simply the medical history that is taken by the doctor on admission (although this is helpful additional information, too, and is found in the History and Physical tab of the chart). Look for the human side of your patient's past. The average patient age in the hospital is about 70. Think of all the life experiences they have accumulated! This lifetime background will effect how we work with them. Understanding them socially and culturally allows a respectful approach to their care.

Simply understanding their background reveals their humanity and allows you to see them as more than simply their diagnosis. Parts of their pasts will also become incorporated into our nursing interventions. For instance, if you discover the patient was a mechanic before he retired, you can draw a conclusion about his competence with his hands. If he needs to learn to self-inject insulin, you may reassure him of his potential to master the skill by reminding him of all the tools he used in the past.

Their past will also help direct our goals. We are always hopeful for return of maximal function. Expectations for a patient who ran marathons before hospitalization will be different than for those who were bed-bound in a skilled nursing facility. It is simple once you think about it, but you need to train yourself to delve into the past and clearly establish the picture of normalcy for each patient.

Another aspect of the patient's past that you need to understand is any chronic medical conditions and to what degree these conditions are controlled. Most patients have what are termed comorbidities. These are not the medical reason for the current hospitalization but are conditions affecting their health. For instance, your patient's admitting diagnosis may be cholelithiasis (gall stones) with cholecystectomy (gall bladder removal surgery).

However, he or she may also have a past diagnosis of diabetes controlled with oral medication and diet. As their nurse, you need to determine how much he or she understands about diabetes, how well it is usually controlled at home and how compliant he or she is with medication self-administration and diet. Can you explain why this would be important to your patient's recovery and nursing care?

So far, we have discussed determining their past level of independence and function and the presence of any medical comorbidity. Another aspect of **Where were they?** is their family situation. Has he or she been married, had children, retired, etc.? If he or she had children, ask about their current ages and where they live. This information again helps you to see the patient as a person within the context of his or her bigger family. It also affects goals and interventions by allowing us to consider resources.

For instance, if your patient will be going home with restrictions on lifting as they recover and you know they have small toddlers at home, we need to address child care plans as part of discharge. If they will not be allowed to drive on discharge, yet live alone, you may need to refer them for transportation assistance. You may discover that they stopped taking their blood pressure medication because they ran out of money last month. The hospital's social services department can be called in to explore resources for financial assistance.

Once you have gotten the picture of **Where were they?**, you can summarize it on the first section of the worksheet. Don't bother with full sentences or complete paragraphs. A worksheet only requires short notes (see the examples of completed worksheets at the end of the chapter). The final aspect of **Where were they?** is to identify what brought them to the hospital.

Physicians call this the "Chief Complaint." In other words, for some reason they went to the doctor. Did they have a sudden chest pain and went to the emergency room? Maybe they had a cough for a few days, but then developed a high fever and difficulty breathing. You get the idea. We need to know exactly what the immediate problem was that brought them into the hospital.

This allows us to understand the diagnostic work-up—what tests are being run while they are in the hospital and what outcomes we might expect. Notice their emotions as they discuss the reason for the hospitalization. Part of our care will focus on helping them cope with their medical challenges. It also takes us into the next section of our patient's big picture: **Where are they?**

Where Are They?

When a patient enters the hospital, the physicians are focused on diagnosing what is wrong. You can think of this first part of the hospital stay as the diagnostic phase. Once the diagnosis is made, treatment can begin (treatment phase). Ideally, treatment will totally fix the problem and the person can return home in the same condition as before the hospital stay. Sometimes, treatment helps control the problem but cannot totally cure it and the patient will go home with some changes (preparing for discharge phase). The average length of stay in the hospital is 3–5 days.

On the day of your work with the patient, find out what hospital day it is and what has been accomplished so far. In other words, **Where are they?** You may only be with them this one day of their hospital stay, as many nursing programs must share clinical space in the hospital and can only have access 1 or 2 days each week for their students. You must be able to see beyond the 1 or 2 days of your care, to picture the entire hospitalization.

Summarize what tests and procedures have been done and what results were found. Has a diagnosis been determined? What treatment has been started and how effective has it been? It is imperative to understand what we are dealing with, so we know what assessments we will make and what observations are important.

An example of someone in diagnostic phase might be a patient who came in through the emergency room the night before your shift. An example of someone in the treatment phase might be a patient who was hospitalized 2 days ago, found to have appendicitis and who underwent removal of the appendix (appendectomy) yesterday. A patient who suffered a stroke (cerebrovascular accident) 1 week ago and is going to be transferred to a rehabilitation center is in the preparing for discharge/transfer phase. Makes sense, right?

After you have completed the **Where were they?** section, and summarized the **Where are they?** as above, turn your attention to clearly identifying the major nursing needs at this moment. This helps focus your care and also demonstrates for your clinical instructor that you are thinking critically about your patient.

In the diagnostic phase, for instance, one of the major nursing needs is for excellent assessment. We often uncover more complete information about the patient's physical condition that assists with differential diagnosis. Information about the onset of the symptoms, what has improved the person's condition or made it worse, any past history, etc., can be invaluable to the physician's diagnostic process.

During diagnostics, patients also need teaching about what to expect for procedures and tests. Sometimes, proper preparation assures validity of the test. For instance, if a patient was not taught why full bowel preparation (referred to as prep) is imperative before a colonoscopy, they may not make the required effort (it is really unpleasant). However, without complete prep, the physician may not be able to visualize. This may result in incomplete procedure or delay of another day while another preparation can be completed.

Some examples of major nursing needs during the treatment phase are for nursing assessment of the response to the treatment. Let's say the diagnosis is pneumonia. This is an infection of the lungs, and antibiotics will be ordered. If the antibiotic is effective against the pathogen (the germ causing the infection), then we expect the patient's symptoms to improve within 24 to 48 hours. See? You are helping your patient's care and demonstrating to the instructor critical thinking when you can say, "The patient was found to have pneumonia, was begun on Erythromycin yesterday and today his fever is down, the white blood cell count is falling and he is coughing less." Hooray for you!

See the examples at the end of the chapter for how you might fill out this section of the worksheet.

As the patient enters the phase of hospitalization that prepares for discharge, nursing is more focused on the future. This takes us into the final phase of our worksheet.

Where Are They Going?

This section is more difficult for student nurses because there is a lack of experience with many disease processes. Consider what condition the patient will be in when he or she leaves the hospital. What will be the needs be on discharge? How much mobility will have returned before he or she goes home? Will there be new medications or a new diet that requires education? Do we need to arrange for assistive equipment at home?

Those types of questions must be answered before picturing what is needed as the patient returns to his or her own world. By the way, although this section is at the end of the worksheet, we do not wait until discharge to begin planning for it. We are anticipating discharge needs from the beginning. But as you begin your nursing career and use this worksheet to appreciate the big picture for your patient, it is presented as a linear process.

So how can you find out what to expect on discharge? You have many resources to help you with this. First of all, ask the patient! Don't be shy about inviting them to talk about what the doctor has told them to expect. This both educates you about what the doctor has said and also provides you with a clear picture of what the patient understands.

Another resource is the patient's primary nurse of the day. Ask questions, too, of your nursing instructor to gain an understanding of what to expect. These experienced nurses can share with you what recovery timeline is usual and what may be expected as someone recovers or lives with a chronic disease condition. They can discuss possible ongoing challenges, other questions to ask or more considerations.

Looking up information in your textbooks and on the Web can help you know what to expect and how to help, too. When utilizing the Internet, remember that some sites are authoritative and others may have an agenda. If your patient is going home with chronic arthritis, for instance, and you want to find out what measures can be taken to improve comfort and motion of their hands, a computer search will bring up sites sponsored by government, commercial, university and private organizations. Government health sources such as the National Institutes of Health and the Centers for Disease Control are authoritative and can be used extensively. Likewise, many private organizations, such as the Arthritis Foundation, or similar foundations for other disease processes (American Cancer Society or the American Heart Association, for instance) are authoritative and can be referenced with confidence.

But be cautious of other sites that might have an agenda or a product to sell. Their information is designed to promote an idea or a particular product and may not be objective. Think critically about who pays for the site, who reviews and assures the information is correct and who updates it.

As you consider nursing needs on discharge, many aspects are easily handled with patient education. For instance, patients often are discharged with surgical incisions. They will need information on handwashing and proper care of the incision site. They will need to know what to report to their doctor and when to return for an appointment. Restrictions on activity and home medications will be ordered by the physician. The nurse becomes the home care teacher. This is one of the most satisfying aspects of nursing.

Equipping patients with information and the ability to function safely on their own is fun and is usually appreciated by them and their families. It is especially treasured if it is delivered thoughtfully, respectful of their preferences and culture and with that degree of human caring we have been talking about. You can be the kind of nurse that patients talk about having made a real difference in their lives. We are helping them get **where they are going**.

Often, to meet discharge needs, nurses involve other resources for the patient. Ask your instructor about what referrals might help your patient. The hospital has many ways to help: diabetic educators, classes about various topics, dietitians, social workers, chaplains and therapists of all kinds, just to name a few. Another hospital resource to tap into when discharge needs are considered is the case manager. This person (often a nurse, sometimes a social worker) is the liaison with the patient's insurance company and can help with coverage for needed equipment or for other ongoing medical needs.

Talk to as many of these people as you can. Pick their brains for information. Find out about possibilities and how to make things happen. You will equip yourself to help this patient and future patients as you build your understanding of resources. You will also demonstrate critical thinking, initiative and compassion to your instructor. Everyone wins!

Examples of completed worksheets follow. The worksheets focus on a man who has had a heart attack (myocardial infarction [MI]). Three completed worksheets are provided. Each describes the same patient, but at three different levels of completion: fair, good and excellent. Instructor's comments follow each of the examples to point out what was covered well in the worksheet and what aspects could be improved.

As you read through, notice how a picture of the patient's situation is painted. You can actually see the person's life. That's what we want because then we know how to help them. Have fun building this into your practice as a nurse. Make a habit of discovering about your patients: **Where were they?**, **Where are they?** and **Where are they going?**

Example 4-1   Worksheet: Where Were They? Where Are They? Where Are They Going?

Where were they? Discover your patient's past and norms before he or she came to the hospital: living arrangements, family, work and recreation. Does he or she have chronic medical problems? Are these controlled? If he or she is retired, what was his or her work?

What changed to bring the patient to the hospital? Chief complaint:

Where are they? Which day of the hospital stay is this? Which phase of care is the patient in: diagnostics, treatment or recovery? Summarize findings so far. Identify the main nursing needs at this moment.

Where are they going? When is discharge expected? Will the admitting problem be completely resolved, or will there be ongoing needs? How can the nurse help to meet these needs?

Example 4-2A   Worksheet Completed by Student for a Patient with Acute Myocardial Infarction: Fair Example

Where were they? Where are they? Where are they going?

Where were they? Discover your patient's past and norms before he or she came to the hospital: living arrangements, family, work and recreation. Does he or she have chronic medical problems? Are these controlled? If he or she is retired, what was his or her work?

Mr. M. is 62 years old. He is married and lives with his wife. They have three children who are grown. He takes medication for high blood pressure, no other drugs.

What changed to bring the patient to the hospital? Chief complaint:

One evening, his chest felt bad and he went to the hospital. He was admitted for observation to rule out a heart attack.

Where are they? Which day of the hospital stay is this? Which phase of care is the patient in: diagnostics, treatment or recovery? Summarize findings so far. Identify the main nursing needs at this moment.

He has been here for 3 days and is out of the intensive care unit. No more chest pain, and his vital signs are stable. Mr. M. still says "it's nothing" when I asked him about his chest pain and hospital stay.

Main nursing needs: I tried to get him to talk about his cardiac status and gave him rest after morning care (sometimes he gets short of breath if he does too much at once). I gave him his medication and he's been a really good patient all day.

Where are they going? When is discharge expected? Will the admitting problem be completely resolved, or will there be ongoing needs? How can the nurse help to meet these needs?

He might go home tomorrow. I called Discharge Planning to get him some oxygen at home.

Needs: Mr. M. says his wife will take him home and this time in the hospital "was not really needed."

Example 4-2B   Fair Example for a Patient with Acute Myocardial Infarction: Instructor's Comments

Where were they? Where are they? Where are they going?

Where were they? Discover your patient's past and norms before he or she came to the hospital: living arrangements, family, work and recreation. Does he or she have chronic medical problems? Are these controlled? If he or she is retired, what was his or her work?

Although this is good information, it is sketchy. A more complete picture of the patient could be drawn if more information was given, and that would allow more thorough nursing care (see the following examples).

What changed to bring the patient to the hospital? Chief complaint:

Again, this is sketchy. No presenting symptoms are given, need more in depth descriptions.

Where are they? Which day of the hospital stay is this? Which phase of care is the patient in: diagnostics, treatment or recovery? Summarize findings so far. Identify the main nursing needs at this moment.

Correct but incomplete information is given. Nowhere does the student nurse clarify the diagnosis—the patient was admitted with a suspected heart attack (r/o MI) but the instructor can't tell if the student even knows that the patient actually did have an MI. Nursing care would be totally different for someone who did have an MI, versus someone who did not.

Good aspects of this worksheet: the student is properly encouraging patient verbalization about the hospitalization and the student allows rest periods when the patient gets short of breath. It would have been a better worksheet if the student showed more understanding of why the patient was short of breath (i.e., because the heart muscle has been damaged, it is not as strong in pumping blood. So to rest the muscle, we are giving oxygen and not working him too much at once).

Where are they going? When is discharge expected? Will the admitting problem be completely resolved, or will there be ongoing needs? How can the nurse help to meet these needs?

Because the previous sections did not provide in-depth information, the student missed some important nursing care needs of this patient (see the other examples for the complete picture). It helps us meet needs when we go deeper in our understanding of our patient.

Example 4-3A   Worksheet Completed by Student for a Patient with Acute Myocardial Infarction (MI): Good Example

---

Where were they? Where are they? Where are they going?

Where were they? Discover your patient's past and norms before he or she came to the hospital: living arrangements, family, work and recreation. Does he or she have chronic medical problems? Are these controlled? If he or she is retired, what was his or her work?

62-year-old married male. Lives with wife who has minor arthritis, otherwise active and healthy. 3 adult children. Plans retirement soon. Enjoys golf and fishing. Takes medication for high blood pressure "when I remember."

What changed to bring the patient to the hospital? Chief complaint:

One evening, felt chest pain and, "my wife made me go to the emergency room. I told her it was nothing." Admitted for observation, to r/o MI.

Where are they? Which day of the hospital stay is this? Which phase of care is the patient in: diagnostics, treatment or recovery? Summarize findings so far. Identify the main nursing needs at this moment.

This is third full day of hospital stay. In ER: troponin level drawn, chest x-ray (negative). Physician's notes confirm MI diagnosis, patient continued to state "it's nothing." Spent 2 days in ICU, now transferred to telemetry floor. No further chest pain. BP controlled on oral meds.

Main nursing needs: give his medication, monitor telemetry, monitor vital signs, give oxygen, and he needs to realize he actually had a heart attack!

Where are they going? When is discharge expected? Will the admitting problem be completely resolved, or will there be ongoing needs? How can the nurse help to meet these needs?

He is excited that he might go home tomorrow. The doctor has not written discharge orders yet, but the nurse says that usually there are some activity restrictions after a heart attack. He will have new medicine to take and will go back to see the doctor soon.

Needs: Since he didn't take his medicine regularly before, he needs teaching about meds and the importance of consistently taking them; MD wants oxygen available at home—arranged via home care agency.

Example 4-3B Good Example for a Patient with Acute Myocardial Infarction (MI): Instructor's Comments

Where were they? Where are they? Where are they going?

Where were they? Discover your patient's past and norms before he or she came to the hospital: living arrangements, family, work and recreation. Does he or she have chronic medical problems? Are these controlled? If he or she is retired, what was his or her work?

This patient description is better than first example, but could be more complete. One good thing is that the student did recognize that the patient was not compliant with medication administration, and in the final section plans to teach about the need for compliance.

What changed to bring the patient to the hospital? Chief complaint:

Although this is factual, it is incomplete: have the patient describe the pain; what brought it on? What relieved it? What made it worse? Has he ever experienced it before? The more specific information nurses collect about pain, the better we assist at diagnosing the problem and the better able we are to meet the patient needs.

Where are they? Which day of the hospital stay is this? Which phase of care is the patient in: diagnostics, treatment or recovery? Summarize findings so far. Identify the main nursing needs at this moment.

The encouraging part of this section is that the student realizes the actual diagnosis of MI was confirmed. The student also recognizes that the patient is still in denial. However, an instructor would speak with the student about how people need coping mechanisms (denial is a coping mechanism for some—a way not to be too afraid). As nurses, we do not agree with a patient's denial message (we would not agree with him that the MI was nothing to worry about) but neither do we challenge too strongly the patient until we see indications that the denial is no longer needed. For instance, often a patient will sheepishly say something like "I guess it was a good thing my wife made me come in." That kind of comment would open the door for further discussion about what symptoms should prompt a return visit.

Another way this worksheet could be better is if the nursing needs were elaborated. Giving a list of tasks does not demonstrate understanding. Tell what you are monitoring for, what purpose the meds are for, what telemetry patterns might be worrisome, etc.

Where are they going? When is discharge expected? Will the admitting problem be completely resolved, or will there be ongoing needs? How can the nurse help to meet these needs?

It is good that the student checked with the nurse about usual expectations. Also good that, because the student recognized the patient did not take his medications regularly before the hospitalization, teaching is planned. The teaching might seem like a lecture, though, unless it is approached from the angle of how it benefits the patient (see the excellent example). And being more specific about which home medications and what instruction the patient needs would make this a better worksheet.

Example 4-4A   Worksheet Completed by Student for a Patient with Acute Myocardial Infarction (MI): Excellent Example

---

Where were they? Where are they? Where are they going?

Where were they? Discover your patient's past and norms before he or she to the hospital: living arrangements, family, work and recreation. Does he or she have chronic medical problems? Are these controlled? If he or she is retired, what was his or her work?

62-year-old married male. Lives with wife in 2 story home. Wife has minor arthritis, otherwise active and healthy. 3 adult children living in other states. Plans retirement soon from public works department. Enjoys golf and fishing. Takes medication for high blood pressure "when I remember."

What changed to bring them to the hospital? Chief complaint:

One evening, felt "squeezing in my chest that sort of took my breath away and shot down my arm" and "my wife made me go to the emergency room. I told her it was nothing." Admitted for observation, to r/o MI.

Where are they? Which day of the hospital stay is this? Which phase of care is the patient in: diagnostics, treatment or recovery? Summarize findings so far. Identify the main nursing needs at this moment.

This is third full day of hospital stay. In ER: troponin and cardiac enzymes drawn, 12 lead EKG done (ST elevation), chest x-ray (negative). Troponin elevated. Cardiac catheterization showed 80% blockage, cleared during balloon angioplasty. Physician's notes confirm MI diagnosis, patient continues to state "it's nothing." Two days in ICU, now transferred to telemetry floor. No further chest pain. BP controlled on oral meds.

Main nursing needs: medications to decrease cardiac irritability, telemetry (be alert for dysrhythmia), decrease oxygen demand rest between activities, monitor labs for anticoagulation therapy (going home on Coumadin), reassure and explain procedures, encourage verbalization. I was able to discuss that when he takes his medication and participates in cardiac rehab, he can likely handle more activity without getting short of breath. "That's good—I want to get back out to the golf course."

Where are they going? When is discharge expected? Will the admitting problem be completely resolved, or will there be ongoing needs? How can the nurse help to meet these needs?

May go home tomorrow. Heart is stable, but complete healing takes weeks more. Some activity restriction, follow up with MD. New medications to take at home. Need to evaluate if he can handle stair climbing without angina; possible to convert downstairs dining room into bedroom short-term if needed.

Needs: teaching about meds, importance of consistently taking them and cautions when on Coumadin; MD wants oxygen available at home—arranged via home care agency. Wife can drive, transportation to MD no problem. Still some denial of MI, but agreed to cardiac rehab program as outpatient.

Example 4-4B   Excellent Example for a Patient with Acute Myocardial Infarction (MI): Instructor's Comments

Where were they? Where are they? Where are they going?

Where were they? Discover your patient's past and norms before he or she came to the hospital: living arrangements, family, work and recreation. Does he or she have chronic medical problems? Are these controlled? If he or she is retired, what was his or her work?

The student gives a more complete description allowing the instructor to actually "see" the patient. Look in the next sections to see how this thorough understanding of what was normal in the patient's life before the MI allowed the student nurse to approach patient teaching within the context of what is important to the patient (golf) and allowed patient discharge needs to be anticipated (i.e., possible difficulty handling stair climbing on discharge).

What changed to bring the patient to the hospital? Chief complaint:

Note the use of quotations and the fact that the student uses this quote to specifically describe the pain. This character of pain, and the patient's denial of the potential danger, are common with MI. Nurses need to be concerned with the description, not simply the presence of pain. It helps with diagnosis and interventions.

Where are they? Which day of the hospital stay is this? Which phase of care is the patient in: diagnostics, treatment or recovery? Summarize findings so far. Identify the main nursing needs at this moment.

Notice that the admitting diagnosis was unclear: "r/o MI" (rule out a heart attack). In this section, the student nurse shows her critical thinking by recognizing more diagnostic tests that were done and following that with the doctor's note confirming the diagnosis. This is critical to good nursing care. Patients are often admitted with an unclear diagnosis (for instance, "altered mental status" or "abdominal pain"), which are really symptoms rather than a clear diagnosis. Once the tests are completed and the physician has determined what the actual medical problem is, the nurse must know what that is.

Also note that the nursing needs are tied to an explanation. For instance, the student does not simply note that she is monitoring telemetry, but indicates her understanding that a person who had an MI is at risk for altered rhythms.

Where are they going? When is discharge expected? Will the admitting problem be completely resolved, or will there be ongoing needs? How can the nurse help to meet these needs?

The student shows in this section how she has used the findings of the other sections to provide what the patient needs. There is indication of cooperation with others to meet patient needs (home care for oxygen) and a referral for cardiac rehabilitation. This man who originally did not even want to go to the doctor has now had effective medical treatment of his condition and nursing care that met his needs and will follow him as he recovers at home. Missing from the plan is more specific information on what would be taught, and there should be teaching on diet changes, too.

Example 4-5A   Worksheet Completed by Student for a Patient with Altered Mental Status: Poor Example

---

Where were they? Where are they? Where are they going?

Where were they? Discover your patient's past and norms before he or she came to the hospital: living arrangements, family, work and recreation. Does he or she have chronic medical problems? Are these controlled? If he or she is retired, what was his or her work?

My patient is a 73-year-old woman who lives in a nursing home. She didn't give me any other information about herself.

What changed to bring them to the hospital? Chief complaint:

The nurses sent her to the hospital to get checked out.

Where are they? Which day of the hospital stay is this? Which phase of care is the patient in: diagnostics, treatment or recovery? Summarize findings so far. Identify the main nursing needs at this moment.

My primary nurse says she won't be here much longer. They have taken out the IV and will send her back probably tomorrow. She never really had much of a fever when I checked her temperature. I gave her the shot of insulin this morning. She ate all of her breakfast. She is a real nice lady.

Where are they going? When is discharge expected? Will the admitting problem be completely resolved, or will there be ongoing needs? How can the nurse help to meet these needs?

She should be picked up by an ambulance and taken back to the nursing home tomorrow. She doesn't drive a car by herself. They will take care of her in the nursing home.

Example 4-5B   Poor Example for a Patient with Altered Mental Status: Instructor's Comments

Where were they? Where are they? Where are they going?

Where were they? Discover your patient's past and norms before he or she came to the hospital: living arrangements, family, work and recreation. Does he or she have chronic medical problems? Are these controlled? If he or she is retired, what was his or her work?

Aside from the patient's age and that she lives in a nursing home, the student doesn't really provide any background information. When you don't find out what was normal for someone, you don't know what can be achieved. See the next worksheet for an example of an excellent write up on the same patient and contrast these two.

What changed to bring the patient to the hospital? Chief complaint:

Why did the nurses need to send her to the hospital? So many possible answers, and each deserves different follow-up: Was she experiencing terrible pain? Or did her blood pressure change dramatically? Or did her heart stop beating? Until you explain exactly what the immediate problem was, it's difficult to plan for her needs.

Where are they? Which day of the hospital stay is this? Which phase of care is the patient in: diagnostics, treatment or recovery? Summarize findings so far. Identify the main nursing needs at this moment.

It's good to know that she is going to be discharged today; but the student's note does not show if she understands what happened with her patient during the hospital stay. Her mental status was affected on admission: what was determined to be the cause of that? Someone who gets insulin injections has diabetes, and that means nurses will be checking other aspects of diabetic control: blood sugar results for instance. And the student mentions that the patient doesn't have a fever. . .did she have one before?

See the next example of an excellent write up on the same patient.

Where are they going? When is discharge expected? Will the admitting problem be completely resolved, or will there be ongoing needs? How can the nurse help to meet these needs?

Discharging to a nursing home is acceptable. But nurses will call the facility and report the patient's status. A written transfer sheet would be prepared, and transportation would be called. These things would be a good to add here for a more complete picture.

Example 4-6A   Worksheet Completed by Student for a Patient with Altered Mental Status: Excellent Example

Where were they? Where are they? Where are they going?

Where were they? Discover your patient's past and norms before he or she came to the hospital: living arrangements, family, work and recreation. Does he or she have chronic medical problems? Are these controlled? If he or she is retired, what was his or her work?

Mrs. Jones is a 73-year-old resident at an assisted living center. The facility is for elderly who can take care of themselves, but are provided with housekeeping and meals in a common dining room. She moved there 2 years ago and likes it because "they take us all over to interesting places and have music every Friday evening." History of diabetes, "My doctor says I do a great job keeping that under control."

What changed to bring the patient to the hospital? Chief complaint:

There is a nurse there who looks in on the residents, and she noticed that Mrs. Jones was "acting different." She couldn't answer basic questions and seemed afraid of the nurse, who usually was treated as a friend. The nurse was concerned and called paramedics who took her to the emergency room.

Where are they? Which day of the hospital stay is this? Which phase of care is the patient in: diagnostics, treatment or recovery? Summarize findings so far. Identify the main nursing needs at this moment.

She was admitted to the hospital 3 days ago, with a diagnosis of AMS (altered mental status) and the doctors thought she might be having a stroke. But diagnostics are now done and the scans did not show any trouble with her brain. They also decided it was not a stroke because she never lost control of movements, talking, or anything like that. Instead, her tests showed that she had an infection in her kidneys. When they tested her urine, it showed that. But she never really had much of a fever, so I was surprised. My primary nurse said that older people don't always show a high temperature or blood cell changes (younger healthy people have an increase in white blood cell count to fight an infection) when they have an infection. Antibiotics in her IV worked great. She's back to "normal"—talking and making sense. Blood sugars ranging in the low 100s. What a nice lady.

Where are they going? When is discharge expected? Will the admitting problem be completely resolved, or will there be ongoing needs? How can the nurse help to meet these needs?

She knows to keep taking the antibiotic pills until all of them are gone now that she's going back home. We got transportation to take her back to the assisted living center.

Example 4-6B Excellent Example for a Patient with Altered Mental Status: Instructor's Comments

Where were they? Where are they? Where are they going?

Where were they? Discover your patient's past and norms before he or she came to the hospital: living arrangements, family, work and recreation. Does he or she have chronic medical problems? Are these controlled? If he or she is retired, what was his or her work?

This description gives a clear picture of a woman who was vital and active. See how much more clear the "story" of the patient is? The student nurse actually asked specific questions until she had a picture of the patient's home life.

It helps to pay attention to the different types of living arrangements for older people. Skilled facilities have licensed personnel providing personal and nursing care to residents who live in a room. Assisted living usually helps only with housekeeping, meals and transportation, but people have their own apartments and independence. Senior residences are simply apartments where all residents are older than a specific age. There may be activities available to them, but participation is optional.

What changed to bring them to the hospital? Chief complaint:

Again, a more thorough description of precipitating factors that led to the trip to the hospital.

Where are they? Which day of the hospital stay is this? Which phase of care is the patient in: diagnostics, treatment or recovery? Summarize findings so far. Identify the main nursing needs at this moment.

Because the student nurse included a summary of what the doctors were considering, and results of the diagnostics that were run, we understand what happened. The student nurse acknowledges her surprise at the lack of signs of an infection, but shows what she learned about the elderly and infections. There are times when a change in the mental status is the only sign of an infection in our elderly patients: look for pneumonia, urinary tract infections or any other possible infection site. Specifying that blood sugars are usually in the low 100s shows that the diabetes is controlled. Even better would be if the student knew the Hg A1c value. Sometimes, an infection will cause diabetes that is usually controlled to become uncontrolled and blood sugars can spike up high.

Where are they going? When is discharge expected? Will the admitting problem be completely resolved, or will there be ongoing needs? How can the nurse help to meet these needs?

Only a few days on antibiotics are not enough to fully clear an infection. Once it is clear the patient did not have a stroke, she can switch to oral antibiotics and go home. The nursing student shares the planning and coordination that helped set up the patient's discharge. Good job!

Example 4-7A   Worksheet Completed by Student for a Patient with Appendicitis: Poor Example

Where were they? Where are they? Where are they going?

Where were they? Discover your patient's past and norms before he or she came to the hospital: living arrangements, family, work and recreation. Does he or she have chronic medical problems? Are these controlled? If he or she is retired, what was his or her work?

My patient is only 13 years old so there's not much to say about his past, he's just a kid. He goes to school and lives at home with his mom and dad and sister.

What changed to bring them to the hospital? Chief complaint:

He was really hurting so his mom brought him to the emergency room.

Where are they? Which day of the hospital stay is this? Which phase of care is the patient in: diagnostics, treatment or recovery? Summarize findings so far. Identify the main nursing needs at this moment.

There's a drain like one of those we saw in lab? The JP it's called, draining some but not much. Poor little guy is hurting even though he has one of those PCA (patient-controlled analgesia) pumps. He really liked it that he could have a 7-Up, he was really thirsty. There is an IV and a Foley catheter, so he is pretty much laying there still so he doesn't hurt as much or disturb all the lines. When we took his temperature, it was high. His mom is there with him most of the time, so I told her to encourage him to drink.

Where are they going? When is discharge expected? Will the admitting problem be completely resolved, or will there be ongoing needs? How can the nurse help to meet these needs?

My primary nurse says he will be in the hospital for a day or two. He needs to get healed up some before he can go home, but he can heal up from this OK. Mostly, it's his mom that takes care of him.

Example 4-7B   Poor Example for a Patient with Appendicitis: Instructor's Comments

Where were they? Where are they? Where are they going?

Where were they? Discover your patient's past and norms before he or she came to the hospital: living arrangements, family, work and recreation. Does he or she have chronic medical problems? Are these controlled? If he or she is retired, what was his or her work?

Basic information is here, but not much detail.

What changed to bring the patient to the hospital? Chief complaint:

It would be better to give more information about the pain he experienced: describe its character, onset, intensity, location.

Where are they? Which day of the hospital stay is this? Which phase of care is the patient in: diagnostics, treatment or recovery? Summarize findings so far. Identify the main nursing needs at this moment.

This student does not tell that the boy had surgery or when the surgery was. The instructor knows there was an operation because of the postoperative drain that is described and the PCA pump. But be sure that you clearly tell the story.

Include a thorough assessment of the affected system and tell what the nurse is doing to take care of it. Instead of saying a temperature is high, give the number. It is good that the student nurse told the mother to encourage fluids. A postoperative patient, especially one with a fever, needs lots of fluids. Nurses use the color of a person's urine as an indicator of whether they are getting enough fluid or not. If the body does not have enough fluid, it holds in water from the urine so the color is dark. When there is enough fluid in the body, water can be passed by the kidneys and the urine is very lightly colored.

Where are they going? When is discharge expected? Will the admitting problem be completely resolved, or will there be ongoing needs? How can the nurse help to meet these needs?

Instead of emphasizing that the mother is caring for him, share what teaching you have provided and what might be expected when they go home. Most of our patients are not totally healed when they go home, so we need to teach them about taking care of a surgical wound, washing hands, watching for infection, etc.

Example 4-8A   Worksheet Completed by Student for a Patient with Appendicitis: Good Example

---

Where were they? Where are they? Where are they going?

Where were they? Discover your patient's past and norms before he or she came to the hospital: living arrangements, family, work and recreation. Does he or she have chronic medical problems? Are these controlled? If he or she is retired, what was his or her work?

My patient is only 13 years old, lives at home with his mom, dad and sister. He usually plays baseball and really is mad that he is missing games (although he says he doesn't mind missing practice). His dad and mom have both been in and show lots of attention and caring. His sister is only 8 and seems afraid of all of the tubes. She left the room crying after seeing her "big brother" like that.

What changed to bring them to the hospital? Chief complaint:

He was fine in the morning, but when he came home from school he was kind of bending over a little. He told his mom he just hurt a little and she had him lie down on the couch while she fixed dinner. When it was time to eat, he tried to come to the table it hurt so bad in his belly that he cried and couldn't stand up straight. "He never cries like that, so I knew it was serious." They went to the ER and he was admitted.

Where are they? Which day of the hospital stay is this? Which phase of care is the patient in: diagnostics, treatment or recovery? Summarize findings so far. Identify the main nursing needs at this moment.

So that was last night and he had surgery right away to remove the appendix. The operation report says the appendix had burst and he has infection in the abdomen from it. There is a big bandage on his right side; the primary nurse says the surgeon will change it this morning. There's some blood stain on it—about the size of a half-dollar. There is only about 20 cc in the JP drain so far; I'll watch it through the shift. His temp is 100.8°F (38.2°C), so we are pushing fluids. His mom is helping.

The nurse says we have to get him up to walk—but my gosh he is hurting bad even with the IV controller for his pain. It was interesting how the primary nurse told him that getting up today will help him get back on the baseball field quicker. He smiled at that and said "I'll try."

Where are they going? When is discharge expected? Will the admitting problem be completely resolved, or will there be ongoing needs? How can the nurse help to meet these needs?

The primary nurse says he will heal up just fine and go home in a few days. But they will have to watch the incision area and maybe change a dressing, so we will teach him and his mom all about that. I was worried about his sister since she was so scared and they told me there is a sibling program here at the hospital, so she will get to go this afternoon and learn about hospitals. That sounds cool.

Example 4-8B Good Example for a Patient with Appendicitis: Instructor's Comments

Where were they? Where are they? Where are they going?

Where were they? Discover your patient's past and norms before he or she came to the hospital: living arrangements, family, work and recreation. Does he or she have chronic medical problems? Are these controlled? If he or she is retired, what was his or her work?

Because the student nurse found out that he likes baseball, we now have something to encourage him to push for recovery. Also because the student discovered the sister's fears, and checked hospital resources, the sister will be given some help with her brother's hospital stay. Asking about resources and sharing your concerns will let you find out about a variety of resources that can help your patients.

What changed to bring them to the hospital? Chief complaint:

See how much more detailed the description is between this example and the previous one? Anyone reading this can picture exactly the acute onset of the pain the child was experiencing and how extreme it was.

Where are they? Which day of the hospital stay is this? Which phase of care is the patient in: diagnostics, treatment or recovery? Summarize findings so far. Identify the main nursing needs at this moment.

Again—a more thorough and organized report of the patient's status; we know that this is the first postoperative day and that the diagnosis was appendicitis with perforation. Notice that the blood stain on the dressing was described by a size everyone can relate to. Another option is to actually measure the diameter of the stain and mark with a felt-tip marker the outline of the drainage. That way you can easily quantify later if there is still active bleeding or not. You will learn other observations that are important in a person right out of surgery and ways of stating pain levels. But this was a good start by a new student nurse.

Where are they going? When is discharge expected? Will the admitting problem be completely resolved, or will there be ongoing needs? How can the nurse help to meet these needs?

It's good to read that the student asked the primary nurse about what to expect regarding the patient's recovery. The more questions you ask and the more you listen, the sooner you will get an idea of what is "usual" and expected.

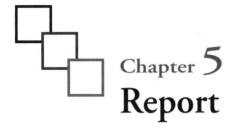

Chapter 5
Report

Typical beginning student report: My patient is real nice. The doctors are not really sure what is wrong with her yet so she's having lots of tests. I've been helping her clean up because the diarrhea comes fast and she can't get to the bathroom in time. She takes shots for her diabetes and let me watch her give one today. That was interesting.

Although these comments show the student nurse's empathy with her patient, it does not present the student professionally. There are more questions when the report is done than answers about the patient's condition: what is the diagnosis? Why does she have diarrhea? When was the patient admitted? Which tests are complete, and what did they show? What tests are still pending? This chapter will help you organize your thoughts and give you a professional report style.

Uses and Importance of Report

Communication between shifts is so important to patient care. Our patients need nursing care 24 hours a day, yet no individual nurse stays all the time. To assure continuity in care, one nurse who is leaving tells the verbal story of what happened while she was with the patient to the nurse who will care for that patient over the next hours. This verbal story from the off-going caregiver to the oncoming caregiver is called report.

You can see the advantage of getting report before you go in to care for the patient. You avoid the need to read the entire chart before your shift. You are immediately aware of the problems that occurred before you arrived. More importantly, you are aware of what interventions helped those problems. Any recent or pending labs, family considerations or important changes are highlighted in report. You get a quick "snapshot" summary of your patients. Report gives you accurate, timely and pertinent information as quickly as possible so that you can get to work.

Nurses have evolved a style of giving report that allows all of this to occur in a few minutes for each patient. This will be an important aspect of nursing that you need to practice and master. This chapter provides a format to use as you give report as experienced professional nurses do. You are then not only able to report to the nurses you are working with, but you will present a polished and coherent report to your instructor. This is a double bonus!

Much of the judgment your instructor makes of your performance comes from these conversations—these reports—between the student and clinical instructor during the shift. When you can discuss your patient in a professional manner, the impression you project is that you understand and that you are thinking. Following a format in your report allows you to insert questions and open these conversations up as learning experiences too.

In other words, as you learn how to give a good report for shift change you are also learning how to communicate to your clinical instructor your level of understanding about the patient and their care. That doesn't mean that you know everything and say it all perfectly in your report. In fact, you may find yourself asking questions as part of the report. But when you follow an intelligent format, group the information you are giving in a logical way and include areas of concern or questions in the report you give, you are demonstrating a very important aspect of education. You are demonstrating critical thinking or clinical reasoning.

Critical thinking means you are identifying important information about your patient, relating it to the physical assessment you have performed, including pertinent laboratory and diagnostic results, and finally arriving at an understanding of the patient's problems. Then from this understanding, you consider what is needed to help and, after providing it, you think about whether it actually did help or not.

This may sound like too much to expect of a student! Yet even a beginning student can use the format in a simple report about a straightforward patient. As you learn more about medicine and nursing, you will care for patients with more complex diagnoses and report will become more complex. But even for the beginning student, all aspects of giving a professional report can be attained.

So report becomes a verbal vehicle for telling about your patient, both to other nurses and also to your instructor. It also becomes an opportunity for you to show off what you know about your patient. A good report will paint a picture of the patient. See why this topic deserves its own chapter? Let's begin by considering what type of information belongs in report.

Professionalism in Report: Just the Facts, Please

There are numerous facts to relate in report: patient demographics; information about the patient's diagnosis, treatment and response; what kinds of medications were needed and how the patient responded to them; the status of any lines or drains; the degree of pain, whether blood pressure or temperature were acceptable; results of tests and labs, etc. The list could go on and on. These are facts that allow the next shift of nurses to understand your patient's status and needs.

We will discuss a format to use that puts this string of facts into a report that is clear and impressive. But first consider that there are some things that do not belong in report. Although it is human nature when telling a story and when dealing with people to include personal opinion or judgments about a person or situation, in report we want only facts.

It takes practice and conscious effort to report factually and nonjudgmentally. But in respect to your patients and yourself, it is a habit well worth cultivating. When you are in the hospital, you will hear reports that include gossip and negative comments about colleagues and patients. You elevate yourself professionally when you rise above the pettiness of that type of report, and you look good to the staff nurses and to your instructor when you report in a professional manner.

Structure to Point You in the Right Direction

Not all nursing environments use the exact same format for report. What follows is a guideline that contains all aspects needed and can be adjusted regionally or as needed to your area and to your instructor's preferences. When giving report, in this order, state the patient's:

- **Room number**
- **Name (some nurses include primary doctor's name here)**
- **Age**
- **Sex (some nurses include race or ethnicity here)**
- **Admission date (some nurses include allergies and code status here)**
- **Admission diagnosis**
  - **Update if needed (i.e., if admission diagnosis is a symptom, and we now know the diagnosis)**
  - **Relay how diagnosis has been confirmed, decided, etc.**
  - **Date of any current surgeries or procedures**
- **Current status of appropriate body systems**
  - **Include vital signs if applicable, labs if applicable**
  - **Note any important changes**

○   **If patient is a recent postoperative patient, also include pain, incision, bowel sounds, mobility, dressings and/or drains**
- **Identify any existing chronic conditions that may need attention**
- **Describe any tubes or equipment and their status**

Do not include:

- Personal judgments
- Your opinions
- Gossip
- Layman's terms—use medical terminology

Here's an example of a student nurse report using this format:

"In room 306 I have B.T., a 78-year-old female admitted 2 days ago with abdominal pain and fever. She doesn't have a fever now. She has had diabetes and high blood pressure for a long time. A Foley is in place. She is incontinent of BM. She is up with assistance. Oxygen at 2 liters per nasal cannula. Saline lock (SL) right arm. She denies pain now, and is still having diarrhea. Today, we sent a stool specimen to the lab for possible infectious colitis."

Doesn't that sound professional? Even though there are some ways this report could be improved, it sounds fairly good because the student followed the format. Can you pick out the elements that the student covered correctly? Beginning with the demographic information sets the stage.

- **Room number**
- **Name (some nurses include primary doctor's name here)**
- **Age**
- **Sex (some nurses include race or ethnicity here)**
- **Admission date; (some nurses include here: allergies; code status)**

"In room 306 I have B.T., a 78-year-old female admitted 2 days ago with abdominal pain and fever." Room number, name (in actual report, you will give the full name, here using initials for patient confidentiality), age, sex, admission date, and admitting diagnosis are properly given. What should come next is an update on the admitting diagnosis. Notice that the patient does not really have a diagnosis, but instead the doctor admitted her using her chief complaint: abdominal pain. That often happens when it is not apparent what the exact problem is. The patient will be admitted and then tests will be done to identify the problem (diagnose) and treat it. If this was the first hospital day, the physician may be awaiting test results before a diagnosis can be made; but this is the third day so something must have been decided.

- **Admission diagnosis**
  - **Update if needed (i.e., if admission diagnosis is a symptom, and we now know the diagnosis)**
  - **Relay how diagnosis has been confirmed, decided, etc.**
  - **Date of any current surgeries or procedures**

The student's reference to lab test at the end of report would have been better to give up front because it tells what diagnosis is suspected: *"She doesn't have a fever now. She denies pain now, and is still having diarrhea. Today we sent a stool specimen to the lab for possible infectious colitis"*. It would have been even better if she had used medical terminology: "She is now afebrile."

Other improvements at this point of the report would be to group all gastrointestinal (GI) system information together. The student reported *"She is incontinent of BM,"* which should come together with the diagnosis clarification, since it involves the same system (GI). Grouping information in your report shows that you are thinking. As you get more experience in assessment, you will also group other GI assessment findings here: *"bowel sounds are active in all four quadrants and there is some guarding on palpation,"* for instance.

- **State current status of appropriate body systems**
  - **Include vital signs if applicable, labs if applicable**
  - **Note any important changes**
  - **If patient is a recent postoperative patient, also include pain, incision, bowel sounds, mobility, dressings and/or drains**

In addition, if the student detailed what diagnostics had been run already, it would have been an even more complete report. Something like: *"So far an abdominal x-ray was negative, and nothing shows on ultrasound, so the doctors haven't decided exactly what the problem is yet,"* would show that the student nurse understood the current status.

- **Identify any existing chronic conditions that may need attention**
- **Use medical terminology**

The student's report gives good information about significant medical history findings: *"She has had diabetes and high blood pressure for a long time."* The reason this is important is that these diseases require monitoring and may need interventions during the hospital stay, even though they are not the main reason for this patient's hospitalization. They are called comorbidities. Nurses sound more professional when they use the proper medical terminology for the conditions: "History of IDDM (insulin-dependant diabetes mellitus) and hypertension."

Better yet, after identifying comorbid conditions, to make a short note of whether they are controlled or not: "*She takes her blood pressure medicine regularly and the BP has been in the 130s/low 80s. Her last blood test for insulin control showed a good HgA1c of 7.*" These are more advanced indicators of diabetic and hypertensive control. If the student was not aware of them, a good clinical instructor would teach about these things after the report was given. In this manner, because of a good report, the student has the opportunity to learn even more.

- **Describe any tubes or equipment and their status**

Lastly, the student summed up the tubes and drains in place for the patient: "*A foley is in place. She is up with assistance. Oxygen at 2 liters per nasal cannula. Saline lock (SL) right arm.*" This was very good. A Foley is a type of catheter that is inserted to drain urine for someone who cannot control urine flow. A SL is a form of intravenous (IV) access that does not have fluid running at the moment, but is available if needed (often antibiotics are administered through the SL, and then after the bag of antibiotics is done, the bag is thrown away but the short line is left for the next dose). It is not unusual for IV antibiotics to be given over 30–60 minutes, three or four times a day. So the SL is convenient, preventing the need to stick a new needle into the vein every time medication is given IV.

The student's report would have been better at this point if it included a statement about what the SL site looks like, since an infected site cannot be used. Something to the effect of: "*SL right arm, no tenderness or redness locally*" is all that is necessary. Again, a good clinical instructor would point out to the beginning student to check for possible infection or problems with the SL site.

So let's put together the student's original report, rearranged for clarity and with the few additional suggested improvements: "*In room 306 I have B.T., a 78-year-old female admitted 2 days ago with abdominal pain and fever. She is now afebrile. She denies pain now, and is still having diarrhea. So far an abdominal x-ray was negative, and nothing shows on ultrasound, so the doctors haven't decided exactly what the problem is yet. Today, we sent a stool specimen to the lab for possible infectious colitis. She is incontinent of BM, bowel sounds are active in all four quadrants and there is some guarding on palpation. History of IDDM (insulin-dependant diabetes mellitus) and hypertension. She takes her blood pressure medicine regularly and the BP has been in the 130s/low 80s. Her last blood test for insulin control showed a good HgA1c of 7. A Foley is in place. She is up with assistance. Oxygen at 2 liters per nasal cannula. Saline lock (SL) right arm. No tenderness or redness locally.*"

WOW! That is an awesome report because the student, by following the format, is grouping information in an intelligent cohesive way and showing a level of understanding about the patient's condition. And yet, if you speak this report out loud it takes less than 3 minutes to say. A nurse would have to read the chart for much longer to get all of that information.

There are other examples at the end of this chapter.

Reporting the Ugly Stuff

Nursing by definition involves caring for people. There are times when people are not nice, when they say things that are difficult to report, or when they are simply negative. Often, this occurs because human beings are stressed when they are in the hospital. Facing pain, physical disease and threatening prognoses can put anyone on edge. And the pathophysiology of some disease processes themselves may cause changes in personality or behavior (sugar or hormone imbalance, electrolyte imbalance, low oxygen or traumatic brain injury are some examples). How can the student nurse report these episodes and yet remain professional? Beyond that, how can the student nurse understand not to take it personally?

When a patient speaks out harshly or responds in an ugly manner or uses language that is offensive, please remember that what is talking is often not the person, but the pain or the fear. There is no intent to personally attack you as the nurse, but simply to let off steam or attempt to cope with something that seems beyond coping. Thicken up your skin and prepare to absorb and deflect what may come. Nurses develop a strange sense of humor to help cope. You may find yourself venting to fellow students or coworkers as your own coping mechanism. But during the shift, in front of the patient and family, the best nurse will focus on the patient and their needs. It is not about the nurse. It is all about the patient and their needs. However, the incidents need to be reported and documented.

Using the patient's own words as a direct quote is effective in detailing the facts without accompanying editorial comment. This is the best approach to reporting patient comments and/or actions that were difficult. State exactly what happened and what assessment findings you noted that may have impact on the situation.

You may state in report or write in your nurse's notes: "Mr. J yelled this afternoon 'Get those #?^* drugs out of my sight! I won't take them; you are all making me sick with those things.' He pushed the medication cup out of my hand and everything fell on the floor. His ammonia level this morning came back very high and the doctor started lactulose. Another lab will be taken tomorrow morning. I have set the bed alarm."

That is a description anyone can picture when hearing or reading it. Yet there is no emotion attached or judgment about the patient behavior. The inclusion of a lab finding that might explain the behavior shows that the student nurse understands there may be a physiologic cause for the patient's behavior. (High ammonia levels can actually damage brain functioning, which is termed hepatic encephalopathy). This student nurse took her report of the incident further to indicate the physician had been called and orders obtained.

Remember: you can't go wrong simply describing events. Using the format described in the beginning of the chapter and keeping the information factual will have you sounding like a professional nurse in no time. However, that first format is not used universally. There are other options for patterning report. One of those used in many hospitals around the country is called by its initials: SBAR (pronounced ess-bar).

SBAR

This is an acronym: S for Situation, B for Background, A for Assessment, and R for Recommendation.

Typical SBAR Form

Your name _____ location _____ date _____

Before you speak with the doctor: Assess the patient, review the chart, know the admitting diagnosis and most recent physician notes.

Have available in your hands or on the computer: Chart, Allergies, Meds, IVs, Labs/results

S = situation   What is the problem?

B = background

Admitting diagnosis
Pertinent medical history
Summary of treatment to date

A = assessment   BP ___ P ___ R ___ T ___ on Oxygen? Y N O2 sat ____

R = recommendation   State what you would like done:

Come and see the patient?
Talk to the patient/family?
Ask for a consult?
Begin or change medication?
Are any tests needed?

If the patient does not improve, when does the doctor want to be called back?

Are there specific parameters the physician wants notification of?

Document the change in condition and the physician contact.

Figure 5-1   SBAR form.

SBAR is often used to report a patient problem to the physician. It provides a format for gathering your thoughts and assuring that you have all the information needed before calling the healthcare provider. When nurses call with all important information at hand, we are quickly able to get what the patient needs, and the nurse sounds professional and capable instead of unprepared or ignorant.

With this format, you are cued to first state the immediate problem, the Situation. Then provide the Background (patient's diagnosis, treatment, code status, etc.). Your Assessment findings follow, stating what the patient's current status is. Lastly, ask for what you want or what you think needs to be done, the Recommendation.

Hospitals often put this format into a worksheet and the nurse "fills in the blanks" to create a report. Then the completed SBAR is used to call the physician or report off to another unit or another hospital if the patient is transferred. Some facilities actually include the completed SBAR as part of the patient's legal chart.

Using the SBAR format helps you to organize your report before calling the doctor or reporting off for the shift. The first format presented in this chapter guided you to group information in an orderly manner that makes sense to the listener. The SBAR provides this same benefit. By filling in an SBAR worksheet, the nurse is guided to organize thoughts and cued to provide complete information.

Another important aspect of readiness to call the physician is to have all of the information you need at your fingertips. The physician will have questions you may need to look up. Having the chart available, or being in front of the computer open to the patient's electronic chart, will allow you to answer as needed. So have those things ready before you call.

Let's take a student report to the instructor identifying a patient problem that needs a physician's input and see what it might look like if the SBAR format was used. The student tells her instructor: "I'm worried about my patient. She only had numbness of the left arm yesterday when she came in. Now she says it is also tingly and numb on the left side of her face. My nurse says we will call the doctor."

The student is correct; a significant change like this should be reported to the physician. Usually, the staff nurse will call while the student nurse listens (because if the doctor gives orders over the phone a student may not receive them, but a staff nurse may). Before calling, though, be sure you have all of the information to give a complete report. If you used the SBAR format to report, you would ask yourself:

S = **what is the situation?**
B = **what is significant in the background?**
A = **what are current pertinent assessment findings?**
R = **what recommendation do I have?**

Answering each of the SBAR points, the student nurse might say something like:

(S) Dr. Jones, this is Susan Smith, student nurse, I am calling about Mrs. Kiley Terrazo at the Mercy Hospital. She is experiencing numbness now on the left side of her face.

(B) She is the 54-year-old woman who came in through the ER last night with left arm numbness. A CT scan of the brain taken last night was negative.

(A) Aside from the increased numbness, there is also some drooping of the left side of her mouth. Other neurologic signs are stable and unremarkable: she moves all extremities equally, her grips are the same as last night (left side weaker than the right), her pupils are equal and react to light, and she carries on an appropriate conversation. Her blood pressure was elevated on admission: 186/92 last night and is still up this morning, 179/88. She has had two doses of the diuretic you ordered.

(R) Do you have any new orders for us?

You can see the similarities between the first format and the SBAR. The hospital where you have your student clinical experience may use a different format, or your clinical instructor may prefer something else. Whatever style you use, choose a method of organizing your thoughts, guiding your assessment and cuing you to share the pertinent information when you give a report.

Example 5-1   Example of Using the Basic Report Format

Take this beginning student nurse report and then use the format to improve it: "My patient is hurting bad. She says she's supposed to go home today but I don't understand why since she still hurts and the urine culture still shows some infection, and she was admitted with pyelonephritis (this is an infection in the urinary tract). When we were talking she told me 'this is nothing new, last year I had the same thing.'"

Take the student's words, put them into the format and add the aspects that were missing:

- **Room number** "In room 326. . .
- **Name (some nurses include primary doctor's name here)** . . .is JP. . .
- **Age** . . .a 35-year-old. . .
- **Sex (some nurses include race or ethnicity here)** . . .female. . .
- **Admission date (some nurses include allergies and code status here)** . . .admitted 2 days ago with. . .
- **Admission diagnosis** . . .pyelonephritis. . .
  - **Update if needed (i.e., if admission diagnosis is a symptom, and we now know the diagnosis)**

- ○ **Relay how diagnosis has been confirmed, decided, etc.** . . . *the urine culture still shows some infection*
- ○ **Date of any current surgeries or procedures**
- **State current status of appropriate body systems.** *She denies burning with urination. . . .The pain is in the left flank. . .*
  - ○ **Include vital signs if applicable, labs if applicable** . . .*the white blood cell count is down some although not back yet to normal range. . .*
  - ○ **Note any important changes** . . .*urine is more clear now than yesterday, after 48 hours on IV antibiotics. . .*
  - ○ **If patient is a recent postoperative patient, also include pain, incision, bowel sounds, mobility, dressings and/or drains**
- **Identify any existing chronic conditions that may need attention** . . .*because she has had this before, I asked her how she tries to avoid recurrent infections. She says she drinks lots of water until her urine is mostly clear. But she "hates using public toilets," so often delays emptying her bladder for many hours. I told her to empty every 3 hours. She also didn't know to wipe from front to back after urinating, so I taught her those things and told her why. "Thanks for letting me know. Maybe I can avoid getting other infections."*
- **Describe any tubes or equipment and their status** . . .*the IV was discontinued.*

Putting it together now, contrast it from the original report: "*In room 326 is JP, a 35-year-old female admitted 2 days ago with pyelonephritis. The urine culture still shows some infection. She denies burning with urination. The pain is in the left flank. The white blood cell count is down some although not back yet to normal range. Urine is clearer now than yesterday, after 48 hours on IV antibiotics. She will go home today on oral antibiotics. Because she has had this before, I asked her how she tries to avoid recurrent infections. She says she drinks lots of water until her urine is mostly clear, but she "hates using public toilets" so often delays emptying her bladder for many hours. I told her to empty every 3 hours. She also didn't know to wipe from front to back after urinating, so I taught her those things and told her why. She said to me: 'Thanks for letting me know. Maybe I can avoid getting other infections.'*"

See how much more complete and how much more organized that is? If you do not know what patient education points to make, ask your clinical instructor or the staff nurse who is working with you. Likewise, they can tell you what labs to check or what diagnostic tests to look for as you learn. But remember that this is an infection in the urinary tract, so the color and odor of the urine is important. Flank pain means pain in the back, over the area of the kidneys. Again, pathology goes back to anatomy and physiology.

Example 5-2

One of the common mistakes of beginning students is to simply list the demographics and orders for the patient, while providing limited information about their current status or condition. This is not as helpful to the oncoming nurse, nor does it show your instructor your understanding about your patient. The following student nurse report shows this mistake. After reading the report, could you draw a mental picture of the patient? Or are there more questions in your mind than answers?

"In room 65, I had Mrs. Jones, a 62-year-old female admitted for hip surgery. She is a patient of Dr. Smith. She is on a regular diet and has no allergies. Her IV is locked off, what do you call that? She is on a regular diet. She went to the bathroom today by herself. The staff nurse gave her pain medication that really helped a lot."

See how you know most of the orders for the patient (these are all available easily and quickly from other sources, though) and yet you have no idea if she even had the surgery yet. Here's an example of the same patient, with a little more individual information; but still not following the format:

"In room 65, I had Mrs. Jones, a 62-year-old patient of Dr. Smith. She was admitted 3 days ago after falling and breaking her hip. She was trying to let the dog out, but as soon as she opened the door a squirrel came across the porch and the dog took off which tripped her, and the fall broke her hip. Her husband is so mad at the dog they are fighting about what to do about it. She hurts but the medicine helped. She didn't want to move around because it hurt too much so I did most of her morning care myself; it was more comfortable for her."

Or what do you think about this report?

"In room 65, I had Mrs. Jones, a 62-year-old patient of Dr. Smith. She was admitted 3 days ago after falling and breaking her hip. They did surgery yesterday and she still has the first surgical bandage on. I asked the staff nurse if I should change it but she said no. I thought nurses change bandages, don't we? Anyway, there is some dried bloody drainage on the bandage. She doesn't try too hard to move around, but we got her up with a lot of help. After that she said it hurt her so the nurse gave her Codeine and it really helped. She has a saline lock on her left wrist and it is not swollen or sore at all."

Example 5-3

Here are some examples of SBAR forms filled out, ready to call the physician. The first example is good and the second example is more thorough.

Typical SBAR Form

Your name _Jane student nurse_   **location** _Security Hospital_   **date** _today's date_

Patient's name _Sally Jones_   **unit** _GYN floor_

Before you speak with the doctor: Assess the patient, review the chart, know the admitting diagnosis and most recent physician notes.

Have available in your hands or on the computer: Chart, Allergies, Meds, IVs, Labs/results

S = situation   What is the problem?

Her blood pressure remains elevated.

B = background   Admitting diagnosis; Pertinent medical history; Summary of treatment to date

Mrs. Jones is 57 year old admitted yesterday for total abdominal hysterectomy. She had been having excessive bleeding and uterine fibroids before the surgery. No other pertinent medical history. Surgery was yesterday.

A = assessment   BP 168/95 P 90 R 22 T 99.1 on Oxygen? Ⓨ N   O2 sat 97%

Each diastolic reading since surgery has been high. Her abdominal bandage has a small amount of dried blood on it.

R = recommendation   State what you would like done:

Maybe she needs some medicine to control her blood pressure.

Come and see the patient?
Talk to the patient/family?
Ask for a consult?
Begin or change medication?
Are any tests needed?

If the patient does not improve, when does the doctor want to be called back?

Are there specific parameters the physician wants notification of?

Document the change in condition and the physician contact.

Figure 5-2   Good example of a completed SBAR form.

Typical SBAR: Better Example

Your name _Jane student nurse_   **location** _Security Hospital_   **date** _today's date_

Patient's name _Sally Jones_   **unit** _GYN floor_

Before you speak with the doctor: Assess the patient, review the chart, know the admitting diagnosis and most recent physician notes.

Have available in your hands or on the computer: Chart, Allergies, Meds, IVs, Labs/results

S = situation   What is the problem?

Blood pressure is elevated.

B = background   Admitting diagnosis; Pertinent medical history; Summary of treatment to date

Mrs. Jones is 57 year old admitted yesterday for total abdominal hysterectomy. She had been having excessive bleeding and uterine fibroids before the surgery. No other pertinent medical history, including pre-op blood pressure was normotensive. Surgery was yesterday.

A = assessment   BP 168/95 P 90 R 22 T 99.1 on Oxygen? Ⓨ N   O2 sat 97%

Each diastolic reading since surgery has been high, ranging from 150s/mid 80s to 160s/low 90s. She acknowledges a slight headache but shows no other symptoms.
Her abdominal bandage has a small amount of dried blood on it. She is on morphine PCA and reports her pain control is good at 4 out of 10 (her personal pain goal was 3 or 4).
She shows no signs of fluid overload: her lungs are clear to auscultation, there is no dependant edema and her weight today is identical to yesterday's admission weight. O2 @3l/nasal canula
This morning's labs show electrolytes within normal limits; hemoglobin and hematocrit are still below normal range.

R = recommendation   State what you would like done:

Would you like to see the patient, or order some blood pressure control medication?

Come and see the patient?
Talk to the patient/family?
Ask for a consult?
Begin or change medication?
Are any tests needed?

If the patient does not improve, when does the doctor want to be called back?
What blood pressure level should we notify you for?

Are there specific parameters the physician wants notification of?
Increased HA, visual problems

Document the change in condition and the physician contact.

Figure 5-3   A more thorough example of a completed SBAR form.

Chapter **6**
Chart Smart

"Taking care of the patients was fine, but I couldn't get over how much paperwork there was!"

"It wasn't so bad, once I started writing something down every time I went into the room. I didn't get behind."

"My nurse said when she first got out of school she couldn't keep up with the charting—she used to stay after her shift for an hour trying to get it all done. I don't want to do that!"

As previous chapters have shown, providing nursing care for our patients is a challenging profession. Yet doing all of the right things with compassion and intelligence is not all it takes: we must also document what we have seen and done. Charting each assessment finding and nursing intervention is critical to being a competent nurse. In this chapter, you will learn what to chart and how to get it all done efficiently during the shift.

Why Bother?

Sometimes nurses get frustrated with the requirement to document, wishing they could simply take care of the patients and not worry about the paperwork. But documentation serves some important purposes and can't be ignored. Actually writing down assessment findings in the chart allows us to communicate with other healthcare providers. Documentation assures we won't forget and can look back and compare findings over time or patient responses to various interventions. Through charting, we are also creating a legal document that chronicles our care and our patients' responses. All of these are important reasons to complete accurate charting.

There are many things you will write about: the patient's assessment, your nursing interventions, the medications you give, the phone calls you make and special circumstances such as admission/discharge/transfer. Each requires factual and clear records, whether you chart on paper or in the computer. Each entry requires the date and time of the entry and is signed by the caregiver, including the license held. Some facilities issue a stamp and include an identification number; but the note still needs to be signed.

Some specialty areas in the hospital use a format of charting special to their patients' needs. For instance, in the recovery room (postanesthesia care unit, PACU) or the intensive care unit (ICU) documentation is very specialized. Student nurses in specialty areas are not usually responsible for charting because it is so different from other areas of the facility. Likewise, if you go as a student nurse to a nursing home or community facility, you are not likely to do any charting. You can ask about and look through some of the charts in these specialty areas, though, and learn something from it.

Assessment

One of the most important aspects of nursing care is completing a thorough assessment, which of course must be documented. A head-to-toe assessment will be completed on each patient at the beginning of each shift. (Physicians call this a physical exam; nurses refer to it as an assessment). Throughout the shift, the assessment will be updated for specific systems or areas of concern. One of your first nursing courses will teach you how to complete a head-to-toe assessment. Basically, as the name implies, it is a systematic examination of your patient. You will master assessment faster if you follow the same routine with each assessment.

Take the assessment paperwork in with you when you do your morning assessment and chart each system as you complete it. The assessment paperwork is usually part of a trifold page which is the 24-hour nurses' note. When you begin your clinical rotation, ask for a copy of the nursing paperwork and check out the assessment portion. There are usually three separate identical sections for assessment: each 8-hour shift completes one full assessment. As a student nurse, you will be responsible for the first assessment of the day when you work a day shift.

If your facility uses electronic medical charting, you can often take the portable computer in with you (this portable, rolling computer is often whimsically referred to as COW, computer on wheels) and complete your assessment by advancing through each screen of the assessment section for your patient. Computer charting usually has many check-off type screens where quick mouse clicks are used instead of marking a paper. Whichever method—paper or computer—the assessment documentation will usually follow each body system.

Following is a sample of a typical assessment portion of a nurses' 24-hour note. There would be a place on the page with the patient's identifying information, the date and the time, and there would be a place for your signature. Sometimes the 24-hour nurses' notes are preprinted with all of the patient information included; other times the nurse will get the form and apply a sticker with the information.

You can see that each system has its own section on the form (or in the computer) and cues regarding that particular assessment. Filling it in as you go allows you to use the form to prompt you to remember all aspects of the assessment. There is also a place for comments in each system. See how nicely that works? Familiarize yourself with the form before you are at the bedside so you can make quick checkmarks. Reading each word would slow you down too much.

During the remainder of the shift, you can make a narrative note if the assessment needs follow-up. It is not correct to chart later on the original assessment section. Each entry is dated and timed in real time. So if your morning assessment was incomplete because you were interrupted for some reason, you simply leave the rest of the assessment form blank. Then when you return, begin a new narrative note (identified with the real time) and finish the assessment and documentation in that note.

Of course, it is important to think about the significance of assessment findings as you chart them! Simply documenting the findings is not enough. When some aspect of an assessment is abnormal or worrisome, the nurse will follow up appropriately.

Task Completion

In addition to completing the assessment, nurses also complete many tasks throughout a shift. Most hospitals' 24-hour nurses' notes include a section that lists the common tasks within a time grid. This allows the nurse to quickly initial or check each task as it is completed under the proper time and avoid writing a lengthy note. If charting is done on computer, there are task completion screens for the common interventions.

So for repetitive actions or recurring needs, the task completion grid is a real time-saver. The time grid would cover 24 hours, so the entire day can be seen at a glance. Reproduced below is a sample of a typical task grid, but the time only covers 8 hours so as to fit on the book's page. The grid on the nurses' note would cover all 24 hours and might extend across a couple of pages of the trifold note.

Neurological	**Genitourinary**
LOC: __alert; __lethargic; __ unresponsive Orientation: __oriented; __forgetful; __disoriented Extremity movement: __full; __limited; __none Grip: __ firm; __ weak; __absent; __numbness Comments:	Urine elimination: __ independent void; __ incontinent: __diapers; __stress foley: __no; __yes; __size; ____date inserted Urine color: __light; __ dark; __BRP, not noted Comments:

Pulmonary
Resp: __no distress; __dyspnea; __cyanosis
Cough: __none; __productive; __hemoptysis
Breath sounds: __clear; __wheezes; __crackles
Location; __R; __L; __bilat; __base; __mid; __apex
Oxygen support: type____; ____liters; ____sats
Chest tube: site(s) _____; type _____
    Suction___cm; ____water seal; ___no air leak
Comments:
	Musculoskeletal
	Ambulation: __independent; __restricted
	    If restricted, explain _____
	Equipment: __none; specify _____
	Bed mobility: __ind; __assist _____
	Comment:
	
	Psychosocial
	Affect: __responsive; __little expression; _____
	Family at bedside: __no; __yes _____
	Comment:

Cardiovascular
Pulses: Apical: _____ rate; ____ rhythm
    Radial: ____ strong and regular
    Pedal: ___present and __strong; ___weak
    Other_____
 	
Chest pain: __denies; ___at rest; __on exertion
Monitor: __on; _____ rhythm; __none
Peripheral edema: __absent; ___present_____
Sequential compression device in use: __yes; __no
Compression stockings in use: __yes; __no
Comments:
	Safety
	__ arm band on; __ call light within reach
	__ allergy band on
	__ bed in lowest position; __wheels locked
	bed rails up: __1; __2; __3; __4
	
	hx of falls?: __no; __yes
	    if yes: risk assessment results: _____
	    extra safety measures: _____
	    fall precautions explained: __pt; __family
	restraint order in place? ___no; __yes
	    if yes: type_____ ; expires _____
	    Comments:

Gastrointestinal
Abdomen: __soft; __tender; __distended
Bowel sounds: __present, __quads; __absent
Date last BM: _____; usual pattern: _____
GI tubes: __no; __yes: specify _____
    If yes: ___gravity; __suction; __clamped
    Drainage: __no; __yes: ____color; other____
Method of nutrition: ___NPO; __oral: __ind; __feed
    __ NG/G-tube
Comments:
	Skin
	Color: __race appropriate; __ pale; __ jaundice
	__warm; __cool; __dry; __moist; __diaphoretic
	
	IV: __no; __yes, site and type _____
	    Site appearance; __ no redness, swelling or pain
	        __ tender; __red; __swollen
	Incision: __no; __yes: _____location
	    If yes, ____length; describe_____
	        edges approximated: __no; __yes
	Wounds: __no; __yes (if yes, fill out wound sheet)
	Comments:

Figure 6-1   Example of a typical assessment form, part of a trifold 24-hour nursing note.

Nurstoons   by Carl Elbing

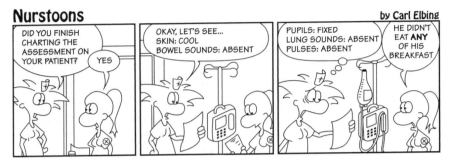

Figure 6-2   (Courtesy of Carl Elbing. Available at http://www.nurstoon.com.)

For most of the tasks on the grid, the nurse simply initials under the correct time. There are some indicators on the grid that are better charted with more than an initial. For instance, look at "Turn (R, L, B)." This refers to repositioning the patient. Instead of initialing when you changed the immobile patient's position in bed, indicate which side, R for right side and L for left side that you turned the patient to. Or if you repositioned the patient so he or she was lying on the back, write a "B" under the time. Since a patient who cannot move independently in bed needs to be repositioned

	0700	0800	0900	1000	1100	1200	1300
Skin care/foley/peri care							
Bowel movement							
Bath/shower/linens/oral care							
Cough/deep breathe							
Activity							
Turn (R, L, B)							
Ted hose on/off							
SCDs on/off							
IV site healthy							
Incentive spirometer							
Dressing change, site:_____							
Call bell/telephone in reach							
Pain scale							

Figure 6-3   Task completion grid.

every 2 hours, this grid becomes a quick record of your compliance with this nursing standard of care. See how quickly that can be charted?

Another grid task that needs more than a simple initial is "Activity." Most paper notes will include a key for activity: "ch" may mean up in chair or "amb" may be used as shorthand for ambulating (which means walking). Nurses pay close attention to the patient's activity level and encourage as much as the patient can handle because of the health benefits of moving around: circulation is enhanced, deep breathing is encouraged, peristalsis is encouraged in the intestines, and the pressure points of the skin are relieved to name a few. Noting patient activity is important.

Notice the empty rows. Most task grids include some of those so you can write in things specific to that patient and track them here. For instance, if the patient has liver disease, they often retain fluid in the abdomen and get very distended. So on one of the empty rows, you could write abdominal girth. Abdominal girth is a measurement of the circumference of the belly at the umbilicus (belly button). Measure it and write the number of inches or centimeters in the grid under the time you measured it. It helps us to quantify how distended, instead of using words like "moderate" or "small" which mean different things to each nurse. Then nurses on the next shift or next day can measure and compare to see if the distention is changing.

Another assessment finding you can measure is ankle circumference. Patients with heart failure or kidney disease may hold in fluid which often collects down in the ankles from simple gravity. If you measure right and left ankle circumference and chart it on the grid, you provide a very clear way for nurses on the next shift or the next day to compare the relative fluid retention. Actually, measuring anything that can be quantified is a great way to take the subjectivity out of assessment!

Here's another hint about improving this task completion grid. For the things the patient does themselves, simply write "self" in the appropriate time column. For instance, many patients can get into the bathroom themselves and take a shower. So on that row, you can write "self" under the appropriate time. Or if they are independent in the bathroom and you are recording their own report about the bowel movement (are you surprised that nurses ask each patient about bowel movements?!), indicate "pt reports 1 BM."

Narrative Notes

Although much of what the nurse does can be charted on the assessment and task completion grid, there are occasions when a written supplemental note is needed. Some hospital policies require a short narrative note every couple of hours during the shift. There are various formats used for these notes. In any format, the idea is to keep it short and factual. As you visit your clinical facility, look up the policies about documentation and check patient charts to see typical paperwork.

The most commonly seen formats for narrative charting are the **SOAP** and the **PIE** approaches. Each is an acronym. **S** = subjective, **O** = objective, **A** = assessment, and **P** = plan. In the other approach, **P** = problem, **I** = intervention, and **E** = evaluation. The similarity is that each organizes our thoughts and approaches the problem oriented nature of caring for patients. Let's consider each separately.

To create a **SOAP** note, first consider the definitions of the terms subjective and objective. Basically, a subjective finding comes from the patient and an objective one is what is seen by the nurse. For example, if the patient says "I am hurting," that is subjective and would be charted just as the patient stated, with quotation marks included. Directly quoting your patient is a powerful form of charting. The "**S**" note in the SOAP format is often a direct quote.

The objective ("**O**") finding is based on what the nurse can see or measure: Blood pressure, pulse elevated. Reports pain 8 on a scale of 0–10. Guarding with movement. Facial musculature tense. Shallow breaths. Notice that in the above example, full sentences are not written. Full sentences increase length of charting and are not desired. Words and short phrases are preferred in our notes. This minimizes both the time needed to write the note and the time needed to read it. Everyone wins!

The "**A**" portion of the SOAP note is where you will indicate what you feel the problem is, based on the objective and subjective findings. Continuing the example above, you might write something such as: uncontrolled pain. Again, the note is short and full sentences are not provided, but a clear picture of the patient's problem is emerging.

"**P**" is the plan and should tell what you are going to do to help the patient's problem. For instance, the nurse could provide pain medications, positioning, compassion, distraction, ice or heat or any number of interventions to help with pain. Sometimes, the physician needs to be called for new orders if previous interventions were not successful in controlling the pain. Indicate under the "P" which actions you plan to use.

Putting all of the SOAP note components together in a chart entry:

(xx/xx/xxxx date), (xxxx military time)
S: "I am hurting."
O: Blood pressure, pulse elevated. Reports pain 8 on a scale of 0–10. Guarding with movement. Facial musculature tense. Shallow breaths.
A: Uncontrolled pain
P: Medications administered, massage provided with repositioning on the left side.

Your signature, SN *(means student nurse)*

If your clinical experience takes place in a facility that used PIE charting, subjective and objective findings are not separated in the note, but lumped together under "P" for problem. The "I" stands for intervention, and the E is evaluation. In this format, the previous example might look like this:

(xx/xx/xxxx date), (xxxx military time)
P = "I am hurting." Blood pressure, pulse elevated. Reports pain 8 on a scale of 0–10. Guarding with movement. Facial musculature tense. Shallow breaths.
I = Pain medication administered and massage provided with repositioning on the left side.
Your signature, SN (means student nurse)

The evaluation portion of a PIE note is often charted later, after the result of the nursing intervention is clear. So about an hour after giving an oral pain medication and providing the other interventions, the nurse would return and check with the patient. Then the "**E**" would be entered, in this case with the patient's own words:

(xx/xx/xxxx date), (xxxx military time)
E: "I feel much better now. it still hurts some, about 3 out of 10. Thanks for your help."
Your signature, SN (means student nurse)

There are other examples at the end of the chapter.

Special Charting

The majority of the documentation of our patients' care is covered in the assessment, task completion grid and narrative charting sections of the 24-hour nurses' note. However, most forms also include other sections for special types of charting.

There may be a section for monitoring after returning from a procedure, since the observations and assessments will be needed more frequently than normal. In addition, special vital signs may be needed. For instance, someone who had orthopedic surgery needs frequent checks of the pulses, sensation, and color in the involved limb, and there may be a special area to make those notations. Teaching our patients and monitoring fluid intake and output (I&O) are other special areas of charting and need to be discussed in more detail.

Key: E = explanation; D = demonstration; A/V = audio-visual; H/O = hand out

Time	Int.	Learning need	Teach method	Applies	Repeats	Performs	No evidence of learning

Figure 6-4   Patient education documentation.

Patient Education

One of the most fun and gratifying aspects of nursing is sharing information with our patients. We teach them about their disease process, medications, any self-care practices that could help them, procedures that are coming up and many, many other things. This patient education is so important that many facilities have a special area on the 24-hour nurses' note to document it. Others use a separate form and include the teaching of other healthcare providers, too, like therapists or dietitians. In the computer record, there are screens for teaching records.

Included here is an example of a typical table chart with a key for documenting patient education. Notice that the format allows complete charting with just a few letters so it is fast and easy to record what you have covered. The patient education chart would be part of the 24 hour nurse's note, or a separate screen on the computer chart.

Using this type of charting, the first column would have the military time you taught, then your initials and then the learning need. Keep it short, as in "diabetic diet," or "infant diaper change," etc. Next put in the one letter key for the teaching method used, or a couple of letters if both apply. Let's say you explained about how to change the baby's diaper and the importance of handwashing in addition to demonstrating how to do it. In that case, both the E, D would be recorded in the column under teaching method. Easy, right?

The last four columns give you the opportunity to indicate the patient's response to the teaching session. In this example, you would either check that you saw the patient apply the information, repeat it, perform it or show no evidence of learning at all. Here is what it might look like for the diaper change example:

Key: E = explanation; D = demonstration; A/V = audio-visual; H/O = hand out

Time	Int.	Learning need	Teach method	Applies	Repeats	Performs	No evidence of learning
0900	LP	Diaper change	E, D		x		
1100	LP	Diaper change				x	

Figure 6-5   Completed sample of patient teaching.

Intake and Output

I&O refers to keeping track of how much fluid our patient is getting and how much is being excreted. Any patient receiving intravenous (IV) fluids, for instance, or patients with heart disease or kidney (renal) disease should be watched carefully for fluid balance so we don't overload them. Others who are at risk for fluid overload are the very young and the very old, so they too will have records kept of their I&O.

The form used to track this is usually kept on the door of the patient's room or on a clipboard hanging outside their door so that measurements can be recorded as the shift goes along. Each time the patient urinates, the nurse will measure before discarding and write it down on the I&O. Any liquids taken in will also be recorded. When the breakfast tray is removed, for instance, count all of the liquids consumed and record it on the I&O sheet. This includes fluids received through the IV, too. Measurements are made in the metric system, so it takes some getting used to. Another consideration is how you actually write the metric volume. In the metric system, 1 cc = 1 mL. Most nurses are used to writing intake in ccs, but when written, the cc may be mistaken for 00. So pay attention to the accepted abbreviations of your facility.

At the end of the shift, the nurse will total up all that has been recorded and enter the shift totals in the chart. The night shift adds all shifts together for a final 24 hour I&O total at the end of each day. As with all of our charting, instead of simply writing numbers, give some consideration to what the numbers are telling you.

If there was much more fluid taken in than was excreted, we need to follow up. Depending on the patient situation, this discrepancy would be interpreted different ways. If the patient had been admitted for vomiting and dehydration, we would be happy to see more fluids in than out since that indicates the patient is recovering from the dehydration. If the patient was in renal failure and had more intake than output we would be worried and checking for indications of fluid overload, since the kidneys seem to be having trouble getting rid of the fluid.

See how something as simple as totaling up what goes in and what comes out is not really so simple after all? Nursing involves thinking all the time and considering what the entire clinical picture is for our patients.

Medication Administration Record

Each time a medication is given, it is documented in the chart on the Medication Administration Record (MAR) or in the electronic medical record. The MAR is printed by the pharmacy with all of the drugs ordered for that patient. Regularly scheduled drugs are usually on separate pages from those given only if needed (or p.r.n.). The MAR is printed from the physician's orders, so the nurse checks to assure the orders were transcribed properly (see Chapter 3). Student nurses often catch transcription mistakes (way to go!). This saves an error and protects our patients.

Nursing students learn quite early in their training about the "rights" of medication administration. We always want the right time, right drug, right dose, right route, right patient (and some now add others: right documentation, right evaluation, right to refuse, etc.) when we administer drugs. Following the MAR carefully as you administer medications will help you perform all the rights whether it is a printed MAR or electronic.

On most forms, the drug is printed on the left side of the page, with columns for the times due on the right side. The nurse charts the time and initials for each drug given. An example form is not printed here because of the variety of possible formats and the common use of computerized MAR. Your clinical instructor will show you the MAR for your facility and instruct in its use.

Facilities with computer charting use the computer as the MAR. Some even have bar code scanning: the patient wears a wrist band with a bar code for their medical record number. The nurse scans the wristband which lets the computer "recognize" who the patient is. The MAR pops up on the screen, showing which drugs are due at this time for this patient. Electronic documentation makes charting easier and safer in this case.

Admission

Another specialty type of charting involves a new patient admission. This is not recorded on the 24-hour nurses' note but instead on a separate packet of forms. Beginning student nurses are not usually responsible for the admission paperwork as it is so involved and is the basis for determining the patient's plan of care. It is a great learning experience to watch a nurse admit a patient, though, so if you can make an opportunity to involve in a patient admission take advantage of it.

Discharge

Likewise, when a patient leaves the hospital, special paperwork and documentation is required. Again, the staff nurse will discharge the patient but participating in discharge is an opportunity for the beginning student nurse. Patient teaching is especially important at discharge. You may be surprised how many forms are required to leave a hospital!

Specialty Units

Patients in the ICU are there because they are more critically sick and need more attention from their nurses. A nurse working on a regular unit may take care of a handful of patients during the shift, but an ICU nurse is assigned fewer patients for safety. Therefore, an ICU nurse may be responsible for only one or two patients during the shift. The documentation reflects the neediness of the patients: there are more frequent checks, more frequent charting and more measurements of vital function. The 24-hour nurses' note in the ICU is more often a flow sheet of four pages instead of a trifold, or the ICU will have special electronic (computer) medical record that is programmed to follow more closely the ICU patient. Beginning students are not usually assigned to the ICU because of the more complex nature of the patient.

If you are sent to a diagnostic clinic within the facility, you are not likely to document while there, but it is always interesting and enlightening to see what charting is done as part of your observation of the unit.

With so many things to document and notes needed for so many things you may be wondering how to get it all done!

A Little at a Time

There is an easy way to keep on top of charting: complete the documentation as you go through the shift. Nurses sometimes feel they don't have time to chart as they go, but the reality is that it can be done if you cultivate the habit. Most facilities keep the daily nurses' notes or the computer for charting right at the patient's room. Medication records are kept where the medications are kept and so also easy to chart as you go.

Charting as you go is not only more time efficient, but also makes charting more accurate. If you wait until later to chart on many patients at a time, details may be forgotten and information can be mixed up. Make a short note every hour or two as you care for your patient and find out more about them. Sometimes the note will be initialing for task completion, making a teaching entry, updating an assessment or actually writing a narrative entry about the patient's condition. The expectation is that you will do one or more of these for each patient every 2 hours, or more often if needed.

Let's pretend there is such a thing as a typical shift (working nurses would laugh at that one!) and indicate what type of charting would be done at each point. To accomplish this, we'll take the time management chart from Chapter 3 and replace the rationale column with one for what kind of charting might be done.

Charting Tips

Throughout this chapter, we have mentioned that some facilities use paper charting and others chart in the computer. Either way, some basic rules apply to each.

1. **Only chart for your own patient**. This sounds like common sense, doesn't it? Surprisingly enough, though, there may be times when you are asked to chart a note for someone, or allow access to the computer under your log on and password. This is not legal! When you log on, you are creating an electronic signature and

Time	Action	Charting
0630	Pre-conference; get assigned primary nurse; plan day	Begin your student worksheet, date, unit assigned and primary nurse's name (this is NOT part of the patient's legal chart).
0700	Take report; complete student worksheet according to Kardex	Take notes on your worksheet from the previous shift (again, NOT part of the legal chart).
0730	Patients rounds; quick assessment; document as you goto assure accuracy and time management	Take the daily nurses' notes (or the portable computer) with you to the bedside and document assessment findings on the patient's chart as you complete the assessment. Interact with compassion and set the caring tone for the day.
0800	Check Medication Administration Record (MAR) with MD orders in chart; Check med box for first morning meds	Some nurses sign the bottom of the pages of the MAR as they check.
0830	Look up any med info, lab info or recheck any assessment info needed for med administration, provide a.m. care	Chart a.m. care under tasks as you go. Also initial off safety check such as call light in reach, bed in low position, etc.
0900	Give 0900 meds with instructor	Chart on MAR (or in the computer) as you give the meds. You can also find out what your patient knows about their regular medications and identify teaching needs.
1000	Make rounds; coordinate with primary nurse re: pt. status. Complete more thorough assessment if needed. Assure charting up to date. Use restroom	Take daily nurse's notes (or the portable computer) with you to the bedside. If the morning assessment was incomplete, complete now and make a follow up note. Other patient needs may include: help walking, reminders to breathe deeply, help getting dressed. Provide this help and then chart it.
1030	Complete morning care, patient treatments. Check chart for pertinent medical history, consult reports, etc. Give report to instructor.	After completing the nursing care, initial it off in the tasks grid; and add a narrative note for pertinent observations, i.e. how well the patient tolerated the activity or social information shared during the care, or pain control, etc.
1100	Take lunch breaks, Students responsible for signing off to primary nurse and patient befor leaving floor.	Before you leave, check your worksheet and assure all required tasks have been completed before you go (see Chapter 3). This is NOT part of the patient's legal chart.
1130	Return to floor. Rounds on patient with care and teaching as indicated. Update charting.	Take daily nurse's notes (or the portable computer) with you to the bedside. Update any assessments that were not normal and chart them in the narrative note. Indicate patient teaching in the place provided or in a narrative note if the form you have does not include a teaching section. This may be a good time to help them walk (called ambulation in the medical field); chart afterwards how far they could go and how well they tolerated it.
1200	Pass lunch trays, assist with care. Update documentation. Check 1300 medications.	Help your patient prepare for lunch. If needed, add a note about how well they ate (or not) and their tolerance. Include fluid intake in I & O (intake and output) graph. Meal times are opportunities to teach about good nutrition (for instance protein needs for healing, or diabetic choices, etc.) and teaching about fluid needs (for instance the value of adequate fluids). If you do this teaching, chart it. These opportunities to share information with your patient are teaching - it is not always a long, formal session. Check your student worksheet for any tasks due; complete and chart. This is NOT part of the patient's legal chart.
1230	Give 1300 meds with instructor. Check with patient for any last needs before leaving floor. Report off to primary before leaving floor. Assure documentation complete.	Chart on MAR (or in the computer) as you give the meds. You can also find out what your patient knows about their regular medications and teach as needed. If you taught them something about a medication you gave in the morning, ask them about it now. Did they remember? Chart this specific learning, i.e. *Can repeat that the blue diuretic pill is to keep my blood pressure under control… hooray!* Check your student worksheet for any tasks due; complete and chart. This is NOT part of the patient's legal chart.
1300	Leave for post-conference. Use restroom. Get a drink.	
1315	Post conference	
	Thanks for working hard!	

Figure 6-6   What to chart—and when to chart.

whatever is documented under your signature is your responsibility. So avoid trying to "help" someone by letting them use your computer when you're logged in.

2. **Chart in real time.** Unfortunately, some nurses chart before the events have happened "to save time." This is actually falsifying a record and is illegal. Or some wait until the end of the shift and then try to complete all of their charting. How could you remember?

If you forgot to chart something in the order it happened, it is tempting to try to write it between the lines or off on the side of a paper document. Avoid the temptation. Instead, simply write on the next narrative note line, with the actual date and time you remembered and indicate you are making a "late entry." Then write out what you forgot. If on paper, use black ink (some allow blue) because it can be photocopied.

3. **Protect the patients' medical information.** There are actually a set of laws protecting the privacy of medical records, called the Health Insurance Portability and Accountability Act (better known as HIPAA). This requires nurses to keep personal information learned on the job private. It is surprising how easy it is to unintentionally reveal information about a patient that should be protected. Imagine you and another student nurse are going down to the hospital cafeteria for lunch. Your friend wants to know how your clinical day is going and is eager to share what has been going on with her patients. As you walk down the hall, use the elevator and sit in the cafeteria, there are many people around. It is possible to be overheard in these public places, so personal names or information that can identify the patient should not be discussed. On the other hand, consider you are at the nurses' station and answer the phone. Someone identifies themselves as a family member of your patient and wants information: "I just called to check on how my mom is doing." The human response is to answer, but privacy concerns limit what you can say and to whom over the phone. Find out your hospital's policy.

Another way we need to protect medical information privacy is to log out of the computer if we're stepping away (don't leave the screen on and logged in, as anyone passing can see private information). Likewise, hardcopy charts are kept behind the nurse's station so only medical personnel have access. Don't leave your worksheets or charts out and visible. It takes some thought and discipline to cultivate this concern for privacy but it is important!

We also cannot discuss our patients with family members when we get home. You may take care of a neighbor, your husband's friend or a crime victim reported on the evening news, but whatever you learned about the person, even the fact that you took care of them, is private medical information and can't be shared.

4. **Do not erase entries.** Errors are not erased, and white out is not used. Instead, any entry that needs to be corrected is marked with one line through and the nurse's initials. The correct information is written after that the crossed out line. Computer programs have ways of lining out entries made in error, too.

How does the saying go? Nothing is really done until the paperwork is done! This chapter has given you a head start on the required documentation you will see as a student nurse. Some examples follow.

Example 6-1   Examples of PIE and SOAP

Here are more examples of well done **PIE** documentation, with the same patient situation also charted in SOAP:

(xx/xx/xxxx, date) (xxxx, military time)
P: Ambulated in hall with one person assist. After 15 feet, became diaphoretic (that means very sweaty) and unable to continue. BP 147/72, P 103 apical regular, R 26. "I don't feel so good." Denies chest pain.
I: A wheelchair was brought, pt. assisted into it, returned to room and assisted into bed. Oxygen 3 liters per nasal cannula started.
E: Recheck 15 minutes later: diaphoresis resolved "I'm fine, I just went too far I guess." BP 138/70, P 96, R 22. Oxygen saturation 98%
Student nurse signature, SN

(xx/xx/xxxx, date) (xxxx, military time)
S: "I don't feel so good."
O: Ambulated in hall with one person assist. After 15 feet, became diaphoretic (that means very sweaty) and unable to continue. BP 147/72, P 103 apical regular, R 26. Denies chest pain.
A: Poor activity tolerance
P: Assist back to room, administer oxygen, rest and recheck in 15 minutes
Student nurse signature, SN

Author's note: In the examples above, the patient's problem is clear with either method of documentation. Notice how the student nurse assessed the patient after the complaint was voiced. Vital signs were taken and documented and the patient was asked about chest pain. And, of course, the patient was assisted back to bed and given oxygen, rested and rechecked in a short time. This is good nursing care, not just good documentation!

Here is another example of narrative charting done well in PIE format:

(xx/xx/xxxx, date) (xxxx, military time)
P: Diminished breath sounds, localized, left lateral base. Lying on left side: "It's more comfortable." Previously, chest was clear to auscultation. Denies cough, guarding with deep breath. Afebrile. Admits using IS (incentive spirometer) "when I remember it." Unable to demonstrate proper IS technique, inhales too quickly, so effort not best and unable to reach target volume.

I: Advised of need to change position every 2 hours, danger of atelectasis and/or pneumonia postoperatively may require longer hospital stay. Instructed preventive benefit of IS and its proper use.

E: "Oh, I didn't realize it was so important, I was just keeping myself as comfortable as possible. I'll move more. But that IS thing. . .I don't know about that. It's really hard."

Student nurse signature, SN

Or the same note in SOAP format

(xx/xx/xxxx, date) (xxxx, military time)

S: "It's more comfortable on the left side." "Oh, the IS? Yeah I use it when I remember."

O: Diminished breath sounds, localized, left lateral base. Lying on left side. Previously chest was clear to auscultation. Denies cough, guarding with deep breath. Afebrile. Unable to demonstrate proper IS technique, inhales too quickly, so effort chamber not best and also unable to reach target volume.

A: Possibly beginning atelectasis left lateral base, not compliant with actions to decrease chance of respiratory complications postoperatively.

P: Advised of need to change position every 2 hours, danger of atelectasis and/or pneumonia postoperatively. Instructed preventive benefit of IS and proper use. Will recheck breath sound in 2 hours. If no improvement or temperature elevates, will call physician.

Student nurse signature, SN

These excellent chart notes are showing the value of the nursing assessment to find a potential problem early and take actions that correct it. That's one of the terrific aspects of nursing: we watch closely for problems the patient is at risk for, and therefore can help prevent the problem, shorten hospital stays and improve outcomes for our patients. Hooray for nurses! You are joining a vital profession.

This situation in the previous notes refers to a patient who had surgery (postoperative). When the student nurse listened to the chest with a stethoscope during morning assessment, there was not good air flow in one specific area (*"diminished breath sounds locally, left lateral base"*). If the lungs are functioning normally, we hear equal air flow in all areas. When one area sounds different or unequal, something is wrong.

A postoperative patient is at risk for pneumonia and atelectasis (a problem where the small alveolar sacs collapse). Remember your anatomy and physiology? The gas exchange takes place in the alveoli, so it is not a good thing to have them collapse! Since the patient did not have a fever or a cough (signs of lung infection, known as pneumonia), the student is thinking the patient probably does not have pneumonia, but may be starting atelectasis.

The note also indicated the student had looked back at previous charting ("Previously chest was clear to auscultation"). Assessment is done in context of what we know about the patient and in comparison with what assessment findings were previously charted. Since previous documentation showed that the chest was clear to auscultation, the student realized this was new and something to take action about.

The actions are appropriate: they target the lungs and work toward opening up the alveoli (use the IS) and moving around the natural secretions so they don't settle and consolidate (change position every 2 hours). The student nurse could have also told the patient to breathe deeply and force a cough every 2 hours and also assure that fluid intake was sufficient to keep secretions thin and easier to cough out. But she covered a couple of important interventions, and if you tell a patient too much at once it is hard for them to remember.

Another excellent aspect of this note is the thorough description given about how the patient was using the IS. The IS is a handy little tool given to most patients after surgery by the Respiratory Therapist, who also teaches how to use it. However, patients are often groggy postoperatively from medication and anesthesia and don't always understand the proper technique. Plus, it is hard to do it correctly! There are two aspects to proper use: inhaling slowly through the mouthpiece and filling the lungs fully. Two separate indicators provide visual feedback about each aspect but even if the patient understands proper use, it is difficult after surgery. So a good nurse reminds the patient to use the IS, watches and corrects any improper technique and also becomes a cheerleader during the attempt. Encouragement is so helpful to the patient achieving a good effort.

Nursing care after this would follow up these problems; and documentation would reflect any changes. For the example given here, the patient benefitted and recovered without atelectasis or pneumonia.

Example 6-2   Other Methods of Charting

Not all hospitals use PIE or SOAP notes. Some simply expect nurses to write a narrative sentence every 2 hours. Often, these sentences are uninformative. Nurses typically write something such as "patient sleeping" or "no complaints." Here are some examples of entries that are short but convey some important information:

- If the facility expects a note when you begin the shift, something such as "Assessment completed" is good (and your assessment would be charted at that time in the assessment section, so even better)

- Social information you discover during conversation that may help with discharge planning is something that makes an informative note. For instance: patient voices concern about restriction on driving after discharge "my doctor says I can't drive for 3 weeks after I get home! My husband can't see well enough to drive anymore, and I always do the grocery shopping. How am I going to cook?" This could be followed with a conversation about other resources: family, church, etc. But if no one else can assist, then we can alert the social service department of the patient's need.

- Another aspect of care that can be charted is the patient's tolerance of activity. Completed shower and shaving independently but c/o (complains of) being "all worn out" with the effort. This helps us track the progress of rehabilitation and plan care.

- An entry could also be charted about the patient's emotional response to the hospitalization. Patients often divulge concerns that may need a chaplain, social worker or simply a concerned nurse's listening skills. Patient admits worries over cancer diagnosis "My salary and my benefits provide health insurance for my family. What if I lose my job because of all the time off work?"

- You can use a note to elaborate an assessment finding, too. If, for instance, you have checked the "disoriented" box under the neurologic assessment, it is good to expand upon what you see that leads you to that. For instance, you might chart, "Patient can follow commands, for instance, cooperates by taking a deep breath so I can listen to the lungs, but when asked who the president is, names a past president who has not been in office for decades." Or you may notice that everyone else is charting that a patient is alert and oriented, but when you actually engage them in conversation it is apparent that there are mental difficulties: "Patient smiles, answers one word questions appropriately and has a pleasant demeanor. But cannot follow a conversation thread. For instance, after answering that her daughter's name is June (correct), I asked where June lives and the patient answered "Oh, she likes pancakes for breakfast." Numerous similar examples of inability to continue a line of thought during our discussion."

Example 6-3

Here is an example of a task grid completed through 1100 for a bed bound. Notice that the nurse does not need to cross out boxes that do not apply. Simply leaving them blank indicates they do not apply.

TABLE 6-1   Nursing Care Grid

	0700	0800	0900	1000	1100	1200	1300
Skin care/Foley/perineal care		SN					
Bowel movement		1					
Bath/shower/linens/oral care			SN				
Cough/deep breathe	SN			SN			
Activity bed bound							
Turn (R, L, B)	B		R		L		
Ted hose on/off		off	on				
SCDs on/off							
IV site healthy SL left arm	X						
Incentive spirometer target 1500			1100				
Dressing change, site:_____							
Call bell/telephone in reach	X	X	X	X	X		
Pain scale	denies		denies				

Here is another example of a task grid completed up to 1100 for an ambulatory patient:

TABLE 6-2   Nursing Care Grid

	0700	0800	0900	1000	1100	1200	1300
Skin care/Foley/perineal care		self					
Bowel movement							
Bath/shower/linens/oral care		self					
Cough/deep breathe		enc.		enc.			
Activity	bed	amb	ch		bed		
Turn (R, L, B)							
Ted hose on/off							
SCDs on/off	on	off			on		
IV site healthy	X				X		
Incentive spirometer							
Dressing change, site:_____							
Call bell/telephone in reach	X			X			
Pain scale of 0–10	4	2			4		

Example 6-4

When you have completed teaching, using the teaching grid keeps the charting simple.

TABLE 6-3   Patient Education

Time	Int.	Learning need	Teach method	Applies	Repeats	Performs	No evidence of learning
1400	SN	Stop smoking	E, H/O				X

Key: A/V = audio-visual; D = demonstration; E = explanation; H/O = hand out.

Since the patient did not show any learning from this teaching session, it would be appropriate to follow up with a narrative note:

(xx/xx/xxx date) (xxxx military time)

P: Leaving unit to go out to smoking area even though he has advanced emphysema and gets short of breath (SOB) with the activity.

I: Encouraged to stop smoking. "Oh, honey, my wife has been telling me for years to stop and I haven't listened to her. Why would I listen to you?"

E: Uninterested in cessation. Left handout for the hospital stop smoking program. Explained how continuing to smoke will worsen his lung disease.

                                        Signed, your name, SN

Example 6-5

Here's an example of documenting a patient who is leaving the hospital but will have to give himself or herself injection of an anticoagulant for a week at home. Since activity will be restricted, the injections help prevent blood clots from forming in the legs. If the injection is to be done once per day, the nurse may give the first one while showing the patient and a family member how. Then for the next dose, the nurse may watch the patient do part or all of it themselves, depending on their level of comfort. It's helpful to note if they do it independently, or need verbal cues to remind them of each step or if they need physical help to actually complete the steps. For the example, let's pretend the grid below covers 3 days of teaching sessions (actually, each would be on its own day's 24-hour flow sheet, but showing them all together allows you to see the progression of the teaching).

TABLE 6-4   Patient Education

Time	Int.	Learning need	Teach method	Applies	Repeats	Performs	No evidence of learning
Day 1	SN	Self-injection Observes	E, D, H/O		X		
Day 2	SN	Self-injection Draws up	E, D	X			
Day 3	SN	Self-injection administers	E			X	

Key: E = explanation; D = demonstration; A/V = audio-visual; H/O = hand out

Chapter 7

The Instructor Works for You!

"I just get so nervous when anyone is watching me do something."

*"I did it perfect in the skills lab at the college, but then today
I was with the instructor and I just couldn't get it right.
It was so frustrating."*

*"It was so neat to hear the instructor talk to my patient today.
She really got my patient to open up and all she did was
say one thing: Tell me about yourself. . .But I noticed she sat
down next to the bed and really listened. I hope I can be as
good a nurse as that one day."*

If you do not have performance anxiety and anticipate no problems in this area—good for you! You might decide to skip this entire chapter. Many student nurses handle clinical performance without difficulty. Although they may be a little self-conscious, they take a deep breath and simply do what is needed. Others seem to enjoy the performance aspects of clinical. Since clinical rotations are the "real thing" the reason they went into nursing and focus is on the patient, they enjoy the experience and eagerly learn what they can. And there is the valuable opportunity to watch your instructor share his or her experience. But for some student nurses, providing nursing care and skills under the watchful eye of a clinical instructor is intimidating.

You are already a successful adult human being; you have made it through the competitive process of admission to nursing school and undoubtedly have many other accomplishments in your life. This nursing education is preparing you for an independent professional position which will allow you to make a good living while being of service to others. You are calm, cool and collected, right?! But now, as a student in a clinical rotation, you will need to demonstrate in front of both the patient and the clinical instructor that you can handle yourself. Yikes!

Most people have some response to this performance situation. It may be a simple as butterflies that calm down immediately. On the other hand, some students are so nervous in front of the instructor that they have trouble showing what they know. In this chapter, we will consider this "performance anxiety" predicament and offer some suggestions to help smooth the way.

Before considering how student nurses can handle the discomfort, it helps to embrace the feelings and identify them. In situations where you are unsure, do you feel: afraid? unsettled? self-conscious? uneasy? For a moment, relate those negative emotions to your patients' feelings. They are hurting, threatened by some physical situation. They do not know what to expect and are afraid of possible negative outcomes. Your patients are dependent on strangers for daily needs; they may have to allow those strangers personal intimacies. Do you think they might feel even more afraid? unsettled? self-conscious? uneasy?

There is value in remembering our human emotions and using them to cultivate empathy in ourselves for the people in our care. However, there is also a need to get beyond them if they impede our progress in school or the workplace. How can the student who is nervous in front of the instructor manage a clinical rotation?

Maintaining Composure with Authority Figures

"Oh, man, here she comes! Why didn't she come when the daughter was thanking me for taking such good care of her mom? No—as soon as she shows up I knock over the IV pole!" Some students feel a sort of doom and gloom related to an instructor's presence. One thing that can help you avoid that is the power of positive thinking.

The easiest way to cultivate positive thinking is in how you talk to yourself. Doesn't that sound funny? But many students who have trouble showing what they know around an instructor admit that they talk quite negatively to themselves. You are not a positive thinker if, in your mind, you say things such as: *"I just never can do it as well in front of someone, especially the one who is giving me a grade!"* or *"I know it when I'm studying, but then it's time for the test and I just get it wrong,"* or *"Every time I did this in the skills lab it was perfect. Then I try it with the instructor watching and I ruin the sterile field."*

These are all negative comments. Repeating them in your mind actually cultivates failure expectations. Would you encourage someone you love to prepare for an important occasion by telling themselves things are going to go wrong? Of course not! Yet some students do that to themselves.

That is the first piece of advice: speak positively to yourself. *"Great! I get a chance to do a catheterization, and with my instructor here I will have help,"* or *"This is a good opportunity to actually take care of real patients. And my instructor has so much good experience I can learn a lot,"* or *"Even though this is a little intimidating to do these things in front of someone, I know I can do it!"*

Another way to maintain composure is simply to be prepared. If you had the opportunity to pick patients the day before, then you can read and plan and picture what you will do to take care of them. Skills that you learned in the lab can be practiced repeatedly until the steps are second nature. Being ready through keeping up with school requirements gives you that assurance that you do know what you are doing. Readiness also suggests having the proper clinical tools: stethoscope, penlight, watch with a second hand, bandage scissors, reference for drugs and labs (some students use a personal digital assistant, some use reference sheets or books). Something as simple as keeping your uniform and shoes clean and looking professional also is part of readiness and projects to others (including your patients and instructor) that you have pride in the position.

Practicing calming techniques will also help you keep positive: slow deep breathing, positive self-talk, consciously relaxing your shoulders, saying a prayer or humming a song. Are these some of the things that helped you before? Use them, or other techniques you know, during clinical rotations when you need to. A side advantage to cultivating relaxation techniques is that you can share them with your patients in preparation for difficult procedures they will face.

Lifestyle choices also make us more or less prepared for handling stress. We all know that getting enough sleep, exercising and eating healthy are all factors under our control (to some degree!). Arranging your life as best as possible to provide these healthful habits will result in you being ready for anything—even taking care of patients in front of your instructor. As a nurse, you will be teaching patients about all of these healthy lifestyle choices; it helps to actually find ways to put them into practice yourself.

Here is a final piece of advice: talk to your instructor. The more you get to know the instructor, the more comfortable you are likely to be. You may have heard from previous students their opinion about a particular instructor. Find out for yourself. There is a boundary; this suggestion does not imply conversations typical of what you would have with a buddy. It is inappropriate to probe about personal things, but quite helpful to ask about the instructor's professional background, training, experiences as a nurse, favorite past nursing jobs and expectations of students.

Understanding Instructor's Personal Preferences

The State Boards of Nursing around the country establish requirements for nurses who want to work as faculty members. In fact, it is the State Boards that establish the laws that govern our nursing practice, set the regulations for education and testing and grant nursing licenses. Each individual state controls its own board, so you will need to learn the laws specific to your state.

Most states require that the nursing instructor have a valid license as a registered nurse in the state and that he or she have a Master's degree. There are various kinds of Master's degrees: a Master's in Nursing, Business Administration, Education, or other field. If the Masters is in nursing, it may be a clinically focused degree or it may not.

In addition to this educational preparation, most faculty members also have many years of experience working as a nurse. Some faculty members and clinical adjunct have experience teaching, too. Of course, all nurses have taught their patients and patients' families over the years, but many have taught nursing students, too. If their Master's was in education or nursing education that is a plus, as they are familiar with how people learn and how to facilitate the process. Many nursing instructors learn "on the job" about teaching practices.

Some of your clinical instructors will also teach you in the classroom (full-time faculty) and others will only take a clinical group (called adjunct faculty). Adjunct faculty members are not responsible for making tests, giving lectures or creating curriculum. They teach their clinical group and do not usually handle the other aspects of nursing education. They may be unaware of what unit you are studying in the classroom; although, if there is good communication between adjunct and full-time faculty this is not a problem. On the other hand, many of them are working shifts on days other than their teaching days so their clinical experience is current.

Understanding your instructor's background, experience and job position will help you understand what to expect and how to succeed in the clinical rotation. All these background factors imply that different clinical instructors will have different strengths and may have different preferences. Paying attention to the "alphabet" after your clinical instructor's name tells you their education level and identifies certifications they have.

In addition to those listed in the Figure 7-1, there are other Master's degrees and other certifications you may see. The point is to look up what is entailed in that line of study or that specific certification and consider the implications for your own clinical rotation. Learn from your instructor's strengths and look to the staff nurses and others for other learning needs.

You can see from this discussion that another aspect of the instructor's different background is that students benefit from a variety of instructors. In most programs, the student has input into the clinical group they sign up for. The temptation is to stay with an instructor who is "comfortable," such as an instructor you have had before.

Degree or credential	Initials associated with degree	Strengths to be expected of the clinical instructor with this credential.
MSN	Master of Science in Nursing	Usually an education and/or administration focus specific to nursing. Well prepared regarding best practices of learning and teaching theories. More likely to have previous nursing experience as a staff nurse or nurse manager, so versed in needs of running a shift and handling a patient assignment.
CNE	Certified Nurse Educator	Must be Master's level and then take and pass the national test that certifies as a nurse educator. Implies understanding of curriculum design, program evaluation, teaching and learning theories.
NP FNP, PNP, WHNP	Nurse practitioner (Family, pediatric, women's health, etc.)	Master's level education plus passing a national certification exam in their specialty. Clinical focus to this education preparation implies an emphasis and expertise in physical assessment, and advanced pharmacology. Many NPs have prescriptive authority (meaning they can prescribe drugs). Not usually well versed in staff nurse shift work, unless previous experience included this level of care.
CNS	Clinical Nurse Specialst	Master's degree with a clinical focus on excellence inpatient care. Implies expert at nursing care from simple to complex patient care. Expert in best practices in nursing procedures and standards of nursing care. This is an avenue of advancement for the bedside nurse. Does not diagnose, does not prescribe. Great resource and instruction for the student nurse.
APN	Advanced practice nurse	Included here so you understand that all nurses who hold Masters degrees are considered advanced practice nurses.
CRNA	Certified registered nurse anesthetist	Master's level nursing degree focused on preparing the registered nurse to provide anesthesia under the supervision of the physician. Not many CRNAs are involved in teaching the beginning student; but their strengths would be critical care patient, ACLS, pharmacology. Not usually versed in staff nurse shift work, unless previous experience included this level of care.
CNM	Certified Nurse Midwife	Master's level nursing degree focused on preparing the registered nurse to support the mother and baby through antepartum, labor, delivery and postpartum. Not many CNMs are involved in teaching the beginning student; but their strengths would be in the OB area and women's health. Not usually versed in staff nurse shift work, unless previous experience included this level of care.
MBA	Master of business administration	No nursing content in this degree, focus is on business. Strengths in understanding of finance, budgets. Good for teaching leadership or team building and nursing management courses.
MPH	Master of public health	This Master's degree studies groups of people and their health, looking at societies and communities instead focusing on individuals. Strengths in medical programs, i.e. immunizations, and other environmental factors that impact community's health, i.e. mosquito abatement. Good for teaching Community Health courses.

Figure 7-1   Instructor credentials.

Nurstoons
by Carl Elbing

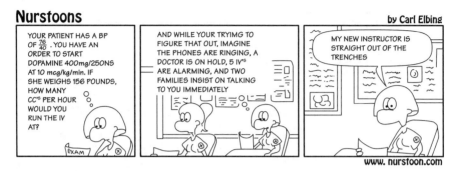

Figure 7-2 (Courtesy of Carl Elbing. Available at http://www.nurstoon.com.)

But taking advantage of instructors of various backgrounds and strengths will provide you a richer background on which to build your nursing expertise. Your own nursing style will likely be a composite of who you are individually and what you have picked up from instructors and staff nurses through your education. Give yourself the advantage of many different inputs.

Giving the Instructor What He or She Needs

In addition to paying attention to the instructor's educational background and areas of experience, the student has other ways of determining what the instructor wants. As in other college courses, the clinical course has a syllabus. This document describes the course: its description, goals and expectations. It usually includes elements the student must show to be successful. For instance, specifying what is required to earn a passing grade. Some programs do not give a letter grade in a clinical course; others do. The syllabus will tell you this.

Another means of identifying what it takes is to look carefully at the student handbook for policies and procedures expected of student nurses. Such aspects as attendance, drug testing, uniforms, background checks, required immunizations, etc., will all be spelled out. Following these school requirements is a big start to providing what the instructor wants and needs from you. Many of these requirements are based on regulations of the State Board or health department or facilities in which you will do your clinical rotations and cannot be ignored. Requirements may include specific immunizations, TB testing, and/or proving that you hold certification in cardiopulmonary resuscitation, for instance.

Each nursing program also has mapped out what the clinical expectations are for each of the semesters of the program. Aspects such as the skills you cover in each level, the types of patients, etc., are in the program guide. Paying attention to this allows you to see the progression of patient care you will be learning.

Finally, the individual instructor will also likely tell you what they are looking for. Before your clinical rotations begin, you will have an "orientation" day. This is usually held at the facility itself. The hospital educator may present the basics about the hospital: where to park, maps of the grounds, how many inpatient beds the hospital has, where to get lunch and such information as that. Some of the pertinent policies may be covered, and the Occupational Safety and Health Administration regulations about training for blood borne pathogens, fire and other emergencies will be provided.

The instructor will cover information for the semester. You will hear about schedules, assignments, paperwork required and a myriad of practical expectations. Hopefully, this is where you find out what things are most important to this instructor for this semester in this facility. If not, ask!

Some questions you might ask:

- What suggestions do you have for us to be successful?
- Can you give us an example of the required paperwork that a student filled out that was excellent? And what made it excellent?
- When we report to you during the shift, what specifically do you want to hear?
- By the end of the semester, how many patients should we be able to handle?
- What specific skills or tasks or thought processes can you best help me with?

Once you have gotten to know your instructor, their strengths and what they expect, share your thoughts and actions during the shift. The instructor will not be there each moment of the shift. There usually will be about 10 students in each clinical group, so the clinical instructor will be running all over the hospital checking on students throughout the day. Much of the time, you are on your own with the patient and working closely with your "primary" nurse—the staff nurse who is assigned to your patient(s).

Take advantage of those times when you see the instructor. Relate what you've accomplished so far: "I've finished the assessment and charted it." This is a good time to ask questions: "But I'm not sure that the bowel sounds were normal. This is the first day postoperatively, and it was really hard to hear any sounds in the abdomen." You have accomplished a couple of good things with those brief comments: you have shown task completion and that you are not just going through the motions, but are thinking about what you are finding and asking for help appropriately.

At that point, a good instructor will probably ask you a couple of questions: How long did you listen in each quadrant? Did you hold the stethoscope firmly against the abdomen? Why might we expect that this patient's bowel sounds may be hypoactive? And then the big one: Is there any nursing intervention you should *do about this?* Depending on what semester you are in, these questions may be simple or may require some thought (this example is discussed in more detail at the end of the chapter).

Another way to show what you know when the instructor is there is to introduce the instructor to your patient. That provides a good opportunity for the patient to brag about you. Most patients are grateful to student nurses who spend more time with them than the regular staff and will express that to the instructor. This is good because it gives the instructor a sense of how you interact with the patient and many will use the quotes from the patient to support their clinical evaluation of you.

Not only do you provide the instructor with information about how you interact with your patient, but introducing the instructor to your patient allows you to observe how the experienced nurse interacts with patients. Pay attention to the body language: how close does the instructor stand? Note eye contact, whether she touches the patient and how information is phrased. If you and the patient have questions, this is a good time to ask them and learn from the instructor's answers.

Share examples of specific things you have done during the shift when you have the opportunity to speak with the instructor. Relating the patient's diagnosis to a class lecture demonstrates that you are applying what you have learned. "My patient today has gall bladder problems: she is showing all of the symptoms we talked about last week. And tomorrow, she will have surgery, so I've been able to tell her what to expect."

Giving examples of teamwork is another admirable thing to share with the instructor. You may have a rotation in the long-term care facility where some patients cannot get out of bed and the nurses need to do everything for them (this is called a "total care" patient). It helps if students work together for some of the physically demanding aspects of care. If so, this is part of what you can report when the instructor comes around: "We have a guy who is bed bound for the past 2 years. He is big—weighs about 300 pounds—and can't even turn over in bed himself. So the other student, Susan, and I worked together on his bed bath and changing the sheets. We used the log rolling technique and even though it was strange at first to change half of the bed before rolling him over and changing the other half, it worked!"

This discussion gives the instructor specific examples of what you are doing, what you understand and where you are in your training. This is how to interact! Remembering that the instructor's job is the assist you to become a nurse helps you to be relaxed. The college of nursing wants every student to be successful. In fact, the college could lose its license to teach nursing students if too many students are not successful. So embrace the clinical rotations as the excellent learning opportunities that they are. You can do it!

Example 7-1

A good clinical nursing instructor asks a lot of questions as we have said. Sometimes, students think this questioning is to "catch" them in a mistake or make them look bad. Not at all! The purpose of each clinical rotation is to take the information you are learning in class and show its application at the patient's bedside. Questions allow the instructor to know where you are in this process, and what you need to get to the next step. Here is the example used earlier in the chapter. Let's discuss what the instructor was trying to establish by asking questions.

The student said: *"I've finished the assessment and charted it. But I'm not sure that the bowel sounds were normal. This is the first day postoperatively and it was really hard to hear any sounds in the abdomen."*

The instructor asked: *"How long did you listen in each quadrant? Did you hold the stethoscope firmly against the abdomen? Why might we expect that this patient's bowel sounds may be hypoactive? Is there any nursing intervention you should do about this?"*

The first questions are focused on how to do the skill: *How long did you listen in each quadrant? Did you hold the stethoscope firmly against the abdomen?* Listening long enough and holding the stethoscope firmly are necessary to be sure you're hearing the sounds properly. If you have not had this part of assessment, simply say so and you will be told how to do it. If you're not sure how firm is firm enough, ask. Avoid getting defensive! Answering with an indignant "Of course I did!" puts off the instructor and you miss a learning opportunity.

The next question probes if the student understands the pathology: *Why might we expect that this patient's bowel sounds may be hypoactive?* It is fine to stall a little so you can think: *"Hmm. . .let me see. . .I'm not sure. . .but the patient had surgery yesterday. . .could that make a difference?"* Again your answer may be met with another question. If the instructor says, *"Yes, surgery definitely affects bowel sounds. How does it?"* Please stay open, as these questions are used to direct you to figure things out for yourself. You can respond *"Well, the patient had general anesthesia and now hurts so is getting narcotic pain medication. Both of those things slow down the intestine."* Yes! When a patient is put under general anesthesia, intestinal movement (called peristalsis) stops. When a patient receives narcotic drugs, peristalsis is slowed. In beginning semesters, you may need to be told these things. Toward the end of your training, it would be expected that you knew these.

And then the big one: *Is there any nursing intervention you should do about this?*

Recognizing a patient problem during assessment is good. Understanding why the problem exists is also good. But best of all is the need to know what to do about the problem. Your clinical experiences are all focused on this. There are always nursing interventions for patient problems. Even if the problem cannot be cured or fixed, we can always take steps for comfort or compassion. By asking this question, the instructor is inviting the student to think about how nurses can help.

If the bowel sounds are totally absent, it is a medical emergency (called paralytic ileus) and the doctor needs to be called. But for slowed peristalsis, there are a few interventions the nurse can take. Actions that stimulate intestinal peristalsis include walking, drinking enough fluids so the stool is soft and moves through better, assuring the diet has enough fiber to provide bulk to the stool so it can move through better and taking stool softeners, laxatives or suppositories to stimulate peristalsis directly. Determining when the last bowel movement was also helps (this gives an idea of how aggressive we need to be: comparing the delay to the normal pattern allows us to plan which steps we need to take). When you are asked what the nurse could do, you would answer as many of these as you were familiar with and the instructor would teach you the others. Makes sense?!

Example 7-2

Here's a word of warning: don't hide when the instructor is on your floor! That type of student behavior sends the signal that you don't know what you're doing so you are hiding, hoping the instructor won't find out. Surprisingly enough. . .it happens.

Example 7-3

Another time when the instructor will be present and need information from the student nurse is with medication administration. This was covered in Chapter 3. It is another time when maintaining composure and answering/asking questions is important to show what you know. There is nothing wrong with using reference books, notes or other materials to answer questions specific to drugs. So have things ready and pages marked when the instructor arrives.

Chapter **8**

Specialty Areas— Avoid Mindless Observation

"Wow! That was so interesting. I knew the anatomy from class, but to actually see the inside of the bowel and what the polyp looked like was really something."

"That was SO boring. I stood on a stool for hours trying to see over the surgeon's shoulder. But I couldn't really see anything and it was so cold in there!"

"I was told to go to the pediatric clinic because the hospital doesn't have a pediatric floor. Which is fine, but when I got to the clinic, they wouldn't let me DO anything except call the kid's name and put them in a room. How's that going to help me be a nurse?"

Most clinical days will be spent in the hospital on a regular floor unit where patients are considered medical or surgical. Because you begin your clinical training with a focus on fundamentals of care, your first clinical rotations usually focus on basic medical–surgical patients. However, there are good reasons for student nurses to occasionally be assigned to other areas of the hospital or to community facilities in neighboring areas.

Sometimes the "off floor" assignments are made to allow the student to experience areas common to hospitals but not often seen by students. Areas such as the operating room or endoscopy unit are places many patients go. Allowing student nurses to see these areas, the type of patients that go there and what the procedures are like enhances their learning. Once the student graduates, there is little opportunity in a busy shift to see these areas. So take advantage of going with your patient whenever you can. After you have spent some time in a specialty area, you will be able to tell the patients what to expect.

Another reason students may be sent to other areas is to provide the opportunity for skills performance that may not be available as often on the floor. For instance, when patients come in for day surgery, they will need an intravenous (IV) line started. Sending students to day surgery allows repeated IV starts and builds confidence in the skill. For hospitals without a pediatric unit, cancer unit, or other specialty area, sending students to an alternate setting geared for that patient population may be the only way to get that type of experience.

Sounds exciting, doesn't it? It is!

Yet, as with most educational opportunities, it will only be as good as you make it. The clinical assignment day intended as an "observation" day on a specialty unit often becomes a passive experience for the student; therefore, the hours may drag and at the end of the shift, students often have difficulty describing what they actually learned. The good news is that you control to a great degree how the experience unfolds.

Seeking Learning Opportunities

Whenever you go to another area, smile at the staff and tell them how appreciative you are to be there. (It helps if you actually mean it!) Watch their responses. You will almost always find one or two staff nurses who are receptive to students (a good clinical instructor will often point out which staff members are usually more open and helpful with students). Understand that this is their daily work setting and if you ingratiate yourself with them, they will help your learning opportunities. Staff members can become annoyed with students who sit around bored and don't try to get involved. Be the student who is open to learn, eager to help and right up there wanting to see and experience whatever comes along.

Asking questions of the staff is terrific, too, but common sense should guide you. It helps if you acknowledge the nurse is busy and time your questions to be least disruptive to the unit's routine. Something like: "I really appreciate you letting me be here during the cardiac catheterization procedure. Please let me know when is a good time to ask you questions—I'd love to find out from an expert what is going on here!" How does the saying go? You gather more flies with honey than with vinegar!?

It helps to immediately set the expectation for what your objectives are on the unit. A good clinical instructor will make it clear why you have been assigned to a specialty area. You may have been given some objectives, a worksheet or a log to track what goes on in the area. (see examples at the end of this chapter). Share the objectives with the staff as the shift begins. That allows the staff to know which rooms or operatories to send you to or which procedures to include you in. You can also gain the added benefit of making notes as you go through the day so you meet all the objectives by the end of the shift.

But what if you have been sent to a specialty area without any direction or specific objectives? What if the specialty area is one where you really cannot actually perform much (like the operating room)? How can you get an active learning experience?

Here is a set of general questions that you can seek out in any assignment that takes you off of the general unit and into a specialty area, unit or facility:

- **Name of the unit/area/facility**
- **Purpose of the special area: why are patients sent there? Will the procedure or treatment be diagnostic or actually treat the patient's problem? If it is a treatment, will it cure the problem? If not, what problems may remain for the patient?**
- **What type of healthcare workers staff the unit and what does each do for the patient? Especially focus on the nursing roles.**
- **Is there any preparation required before the patient goes to the unit? Does a nurse assist this preparation? How?**
- **What does the experience feel like to the patient?**
- **What will happen after the patient leaves the area? What are the nursing responsibilities, if any, afterwards?**
- **Note any specific tasks you were able to perform for the patient while on the unit.**

Using these guiding questions, let's see how a student nurse completed it to reflect a day in the Endoscopy Clinic.

- **Name of the unit.** Endoscopy clinic
- **Purpose of the special area: why are patients sent there? Will the procedure or treatment be diagnostic or actually treat the patient's problem? If it is a treatment, will it cure the problem? If not, what problems may remain for the patient?** Patients are sent to the endoscopy area for scope procedures. That means the physician passes a tube into the gastrointestinal (GI) tract to see what's inside. They can go down the esophagus and look at the top of the GI tract, or put the tube up into the colon and see inside the intestine. Seeing the inside lets the doctor see if it is normal or not, and sometimes what's causing the patient

problems like nausea, bleeding or pain. The nurses here told me that they do some other procedures sometimes (like put in a G-tube for feedings directly into the stomach, but I didn't see any of those.)

Sometimes they do diagnostic procedures (like taking biopsy samples of polyps or ulcer areas). But it can also be a treatment, like the one colonoscopy I watched where they found two hemorrhoids that were bleeding. They took them out right then and there. And of course, colonoscopy is also a screening procedure to be sure that someone doesn't have cancer or something. I remember in class that we were told everyone over 50 years old should get a colonoscopy every 5 years, or 10 years or something.

For this patient, since the hemorrhoids were removed, they will not be there to bleed again. But she is at risk to get more of them if she doesn't keep her stools soft and moving each day. For some other people, the scope procedure might not totally take care of the problem. If they found a cancer tumor, then there would be treatment after the scope. If they found other disease, the patient might need medicine or surgery or a new diet or something else.

- **What type of healthcare workers staff the unit and what does each do for the patient? Especially focus on the nursing roles.** There was a doctor in one of the rooms, and a physician's assistant (PA) in the other. They told me a PA has a master's degree. This woman did the routine scope procedures and could ask the physician if something came up. I was surprised that the PA gave drugs and orders for the sedation just like the doctor did.

  They had a tech to clean the scopes and set up the rooms before the patient came. He also moved the patient around on the table during the scope so the tube could pass and the doctor could see well.

  There were nurses, too, who got the patients ready and then stayed in the room to give the IV sedation drugs and watch out for the patient. The nurse I worked with was awesome. This one patient was nervous, saying how undignified it seemed to have people "looking up her rear end." The nurse held her hand and smiled and said how they just wanted to make her better (this lady was having blood in her stools). I saw how the nurse's attention and attitude eased the lady. After it was done, the patient squeezed the nurse's hand and thanked her for helping. It was nice to see; I mean the nurse was just being nice, not a big deal, but the patient really was touched. I liked that.

- **Is there any preparation required before the patient goes to the unit? Does a nurse assist this preparation? How?** This lady came in from home (some of the patients came in from the hospital), so she did her own preparation for the colonos-copy. I asked her about it and she made a face and told me it was awful. She had to take laxative pills and told me she had to drink gallons of an icky kind of water that made her go and go until all that came out after hours was not stool any more but just liquid. Ugh. Not that it hurt or anything. Oh, and she couldn't eat or drink anything the whole night before. But she said it made sense since they had to clean out everything so they would be able to see what was going on up there. If the patient is in the hospital before the procedure, the staff nurses would be sure that same kind of preparation was done.

- **What does the experience feel like to the patient?** When she first came in, the lady was a little shaky and we helped her get onto the table. The preparation made her a little weak. I watched the nurse start the IV and once she had some medication in the IV, she really didn't seem to know about anything (I mean she didn't make a face of groan or anything). After it was done, she had so much loud gas that she blushed and kept saying excuse me. But the nurse told her it was good that she was getting all of that out. When they had the scope in her, they pushed gas in to open up the walls of the intestine so they could see better. Of course she had gas after! And even though the nurse was gentle and nice to her, the patient said when she left about how she hopes it's a long time before she needs to go through that again. I think she was still a little embarrassed about the whole thing.

- **What will happen after the patient leaves the area? What are the nursing responsibilities, if any, afterwards?** The doctor told her she might have some more streaks of blood with stool a few days as the area heals where he removed the hemorrhoid. The nurse gave her information about how to eat and drink to keep the stool soft so she doesn't get hemorrhoids again. It will be important for her not to strain or push hard to get the stool out.

- **Note any specific tasks you were able to perform for the patient while on the unit.** I wanted to start the IV on her when she first came, but she is an older lady with small veins and the preparation made her a little dehydrated, so the nurse said to just watch this time. Two patients who later came in had good veins and I started both IVs! The first guy had rolling veins and I had to stick him twice. He was nice, but I felt bad to have to try twice. The nurse showed me how to pull down with my thumb to kind of anchor the vein before I pushed the needle in and I got it! It was cool. I also made the patients feel comfortable and enjoyed talking to them before the doctor did the procedure. It's fun to get to know the patients.

See how using the guideline questions help you to focus your experience and look for certain things, instead of just passively watching?

Skill Performance Successfully

Part of your training as a nurse involves mastering technical skills such as taking vital signs (VS), starting an IV, inserting catheters, etc. These will be taught in a lab class and practiced first on other students, family members or manikins. Some manikins are quite sophisticated and include computers inside that simulate breath sounds and heart rhythms, etc. But during your clinical days, you get an opportunity to perform these skills for real people. Completing skills successfully with patients is often a nervous experience for students. Here are some ideas to make it easier and allow you to successfully complete skills in the hospital with your instructor supervising.

The best advice is to be prepared. Any skill needs practice.

Think back to when you learned to drive a car. There seemed to be so many different things to think about at one time: the pedals for acceleration or braking, steering while judging where the car was in the lane, checking the mirrors, looking at the dials and gauges, not to mention trying to park. And yet now you don't give a second thought to most actions involved in driving. You simply get in and go. What created the mastery of the skill? Practice.

When someone gets so practiced that actions are taken without thinking, it is called automaticity. That's a fancy word for the recognition that, if you do something many times, you eventually stop thinking about each individual step. The hope for your nursing skills is that you will take many of them to the level of automaticity. It just takes practice. Nursing school includes practice time in lab classes, but you will master skills more quickly if you practice on your own too. Then when you are in the hospital on a clinical day, skills performance will not be quite as scary because each step has been done many times.

It is different of course to perform a skill on a real person, though. And the opportunity for skills often comes when you are assigned to a specialty unit. So, let's say you are quite comfortable doing the skill in the lab or for a fellow student and now it is a clinical day and you are preparing to perform the skill while your instructor supervises.

Successful Skills Performance on REAL patients with your Clinical Instructor present

1. Assess your patient for the skill; get permission
2. Plan what you will do
   • Review in your head what you learned in the lab
   • Look up the Policy and Procedure, compare
   • Gather supplies
   • Meet with your clinical instructor and discuss the skill; talk through it; discuss any differences in how you learned it and what this hospital's policy and procedure is
3. Go to the patient's room
   • Introduce your instructor
   • Perform the skill! Way to go!
4. After completion, make note of what you did well. Then consider anything you will do differently next time. Ask for feedback from your instructor.

Figure 8-1   Successful skills performance on real patients with your clinical instructor present.

Let's look at each step:

1. **Assess your patient for the skill; get permission**

   Before "just doing" the skill, check first that this patient presents a good practice opportunity for you. Let's say you are in the day surgery department, you have identified to the staff that you want to get chances to start IVs and the primary nurse tells you the patient in the next room needs an IV started! Introduce yourself to the patient as a student nurse and, with a smile and some confidence, offer that you would like to check for good IV start sites.

   Then wrap the tourniquet and take your time checking for a good vein. When you are new at IV starts, you are more likely to be successful if you pick someone with good veins. Make it easy! The vein should feel elastic and full under your fingers, with a bit of a bounce. If you don't feel a good one, move around the arm and/or check the other arm. Spending time assessing for a good vein is well worth it. If you only feel very small veins, the patient has lots of bruising or you can't feel a good vein—don't ask to try on that patient.

   If you feel a good vein (and the primary nurse can help with this assessment; sometimes the patient even knows where they have a "good" vein), then ask the patient's permission to start the IV. Your thorough assessment has likely reassured them that you are careful. You can also reassure that your instructor (or the primary nurse) will be with you to help things go well. It is humbling to see how willing patients are to allow themselves to be "guinea pigs" for student practice. The patient usually agrees and says something such as, "Everyone has to learn sometime." It helps if you *don't* announce with trembling voice, "You would be my first real IV start." Just say how much you have prepared and practiced and that you will do your very best. Then tell him or her you will get ready and return.

2. **Plan what you will do**
   - **Review in your head what you learned in the lab: think positively!**
   - **Look up the Policy and Procedure, compare**
   - **Gather supplies**
   - **Meet with your clinical instructor and discuss the skill; talk through it; discuss any differences in how you learned it and what this hospital's policy and procedure is**

   Leave the patient's bedside and get yourself ready. This involves some positive self-talk. Remind yourself how well you did in skills lab, and that you are going to do just fine. Think of how you would encourage your best friend or your child if they were about to face a challenge. Treat yourself just as well: "I can do this!"

   Look up the Policy and Procedure for the skill you are going to perform and check that the hospital's procedure matches what you were taught. Sometimes, there are minor differences that you must follow. Go through the steps in your mind or with the primary nurse or another student. Practice mentally what you practiced in the lab.

Gather your supplies together and call your instructor. Take time to talk through the steps with your instructor before you get to the patient's room. Ask if the clinical instructor has any specific suggestions for you before you start (you may get some good tips!). This ends your practice and you are ready to head for the patient's room.

3. **Go to the patient's room**
   - **Introduce your instructor**
   - **Perform the skill! Way to go!**

Once you are at the bedside, introduce your instructor and, with a smile, set up your supplies close to where you will be working. Be sure you have good light and that there are not distractions (for instance, turn off the TV, close the door, etc.). Wash your hands, put on gloves, wrap the tourniquet, point out to your instructor which vein you have chosen, prepare the skin, take a steady breath and pierce into the vein. Follow the steps you have learned to secure the catheter and dress the site. Hooray! You have started your first IV! Smile and thank the patient, clean up the area and leave the room, glowing with success.

4. **After completion, make note of what you did well. Then consider anything you will do differently next time. Ask for feedback from your instructor.**

Students are sometimes surprised by getting shaky *after* they have completed a skill, but it often happens. You concentrate so hard and require "professional" behavior in front of the patient that sometimes there is a let down afterwards. That is fine. Give yourself a minute and, again, enjoy some positive talk for yourself.

Even if you were not totally successful in the skill performance, maybe you needed some help from the instructor or primary nurse to complete the skill; there are always aspects you did well. Take time first to focus on what you did correctly. This is important and not simply a psychologic trick. Recognizing the steps we did well allows us to repeat them. Students tend to be too critical, often ignoring the many things they did well. It is difficult to repeat success if you don't recognize it! So remind yourself first of each step you did well during the skill performance.

Equally important is to recognize ways you can improve next time. Technically, maybe you can hold your equipment differently, approach the skin at a different angle, or have your supplies closer to you, etc. Ask your instructor for recommendations for performance improvement. The entire point of taking clinical courses and actually caring for people in the hospital is to practice and learn. If we could do it perfectly without practice, we would never be students. Everyone can improve. Listen openly to suggestions and try not to get defensive.

Skills Performance: More Than a Technical Exercise

So far, we have focused on the technical task completion aspect of skills performance. However, consider that the procedure is being done for a human being! This person has feelings and fears. Performing a skill requires the student nurse remember the human needs, too. Our patients are often afraid and/or hurting and may be fearful of what you are going to do. They need reassurance and compassion.

Because this is a human being and not the skills lab manikin, your approach and treatment of the patient during skills performance is important. At first, it is difficult to focus on the patient because you are thinking so hard about the steps involved. You might even let the patient know beforehand, with a smile and a pat or hug that you care about them and understand this may be uncomfortable for them and that although it may seem that you are ignoring them during the skill performance, you are concentrating hard to do a good job. As you get more practiced, you will get to a point where you can pay attention to the patient's response during skills and adjust what you're doing depending on them. But one step at a time!

The other aspect of skills performance that goes beyond the task itself is the reason behind the procedure. A nurse needs to know why a procedure or skill is being done: how will it benefit the patient? Will it give us information or will it correct a problem? For instance, an IV may be ordered for many different reasons. Our example of the patient in the day surgery is having an IV started so drugs can be administered to control anesthesia or as a route for emergency response in case it becomes necessary. Yet IVs can also deliver drugs or provide fluids, depending on the patient needs. See how there is thought and expectation behind the skill itself?

This aspect of understanding the clinical reasoning behind the skill performance is important, too. Consider *why* a skill was ordered; share with the person how the procedure will help them. As a patient, it is much easier to tolerate an uncomfortable procedure if you understand how it benefits you. As a student, it is clearer what to watch for and follow-up on if you appreciate why the procedure/skill was needed.

Following up our IV start example: if the person was dehydrated and needed the IV to get fluids back into them, then the student who understands that will be watching for signs that the body is getting a better fluid balance (urine will get lighter in color, skin will not be so dry, if eyes were sunken they will be less so, there may be increases in blood pressure, etc.). If the person needed the IV for antibiotics to fight an infection, then the student nurse will watch for a decrease in temperature, decrease in white blood cells in the lab reports and visible signs wherever the infection site was of improvements (for instance, less drainage of the wound or, if the infection was in the lungs, clearer sputum, etc.). See how it makes sense? The reason for starting the IV (or for doing any other procedure) guides the nurse's follow-up assessment to assure the desired outcome is being achieved.

When you can complete the skill, consider the patient's comfort and understand the reason for the skill in the first place—you are on your way to becoming a nurse!

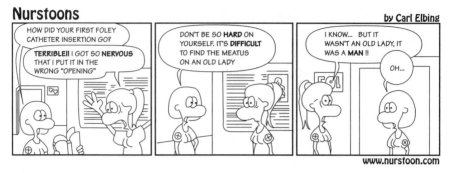

Figure 8-2   (Courtesy of Carl Elbing. Available at www.nurstoon.com.)

Code Blue!

When a patient has no pulse, no breathing and/or is unresponsive, the nurse begins basic life support and calls for help. A prerequisite to nursing school admission usually includes completion of a basic life support course. You likely have a cardiopulmonary resuscitation (CPR) card; if not, it is highly recommended. The American Heart Association offers courses regularly in most communities. This course will prepare you to recognize when a person needs resuscitation, know how to call to activate emergency responders, to begin compressions and rescue breathing and to apply and use an external defibrillator. This type of response is used in a hospital setting also. Beyond the basics of CPR, the hospital also has a team of people who take basic life support to the next level to save a patient's life. It is common to call this a Code Blue situation, and to refer to the responding team as the Code Team.

If a code is called when you are in the facility, be sure to go! You can be one of the people who provide compressions. This allows you to be right up with the patient and the Code Team and see what goes on. The first time you are involved in a code response, it may seem quite chaotic. There is quite a bit of simultaneous action, but all of it is well planned. Thinking about it ahead of time, and picturing "who does what" will allow you to watch for and participate in responder positions and roles during the real thing (see Anatomy of a Code in Figs. 8-3 and 8-4).

Staff Nurses Are Lifesavers

The first nurse in the room identifying the unresponsiveness of the patient starts the code response. She will yell loudly for help (or push the "code button" on the wall if the room has it) while opening the patient's airway and checking for breathing. If the patient is not breathing, she provides rescue breaths with a barrier device. If there is no pulse, she will put a backboard under the patient and begin compressions. On most

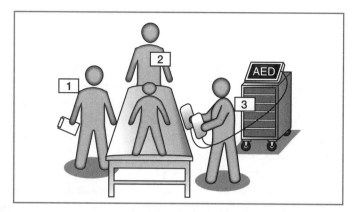

Figure 8-3   Anatomy of a code—staff nurse response.

- The first three nurses begin the code response (see pages 136 and 138).

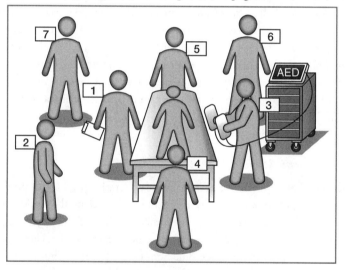

Figure 8-4   Code team arrives.

- 4 – Team leader – this is the physician who calls the orders and runs the code.
- 5 – Anesthesiologist or respiratory therapist – this person will take over at the head; relieve the nurse who was providing breaths. They will intubate and use Ambu bag to support respirations. Sometimes they are responsible for getting blood gasses; other places the lab people do this.
- 6 – Intensive care nurse – or other ACLS (Advanced Cardiac Life Support) certified nurse will administer drugs from the crash cart per the algorithm of ACLS, and/or the physician's orders
- 7 – other responders may come, see chapter for discussion

hospital beds, the headboard pulls right out and can be used as a backboard. Other, newer beds have a handle to pull specifically for CPR that makes the bed firm and brings it up to the responders' level.

The second nurse arriving takes over breathing and the two nurses continue CPR until the crash cart arrives. Each hospital unit has at least one crash cart: a rolling cart with all the supplies needed for code response. One of the things you will learn as a student nurse is where the carts are kept and which drawers hold which supplies.

As soon as the crash cart arrives (usually within minutes of the first nurse finding the patient), apply the defibrillator pads and check for the cardiac rhythm. Most adults go down because of cardiac arrest or a fatal arrhythmia. Their survival chance is greatly increased by quick defibrillation (shock) that the automatic external defibrillator (AED) provides. Notice that all of this response has happened within just a few minutes and before any of the Code Team arrives. Nurses on the floor are lifesavers!

As the crash cart is brought in the room, usually other nurses come too because they know you need help. One of these nurses will become the recorder. The recording nurse writes down minute by minute what happens in a code response. There is a form specifically for this purpose and it is usually located on the outside of the crash cart. The code form becomes the nurses' notes and doctor's orders, so it is a very important piece of paper. Other nurses may start an IV if there is not one, move furniture out of the way to make room for the team or set up the airway equipment, and take care of the family members.

The Code Team Arrives

The exact members of the code team may vary from hospital to hospital. In some places, the emergency room (ER) physicians and personnel are the Code Team for the hospital. Other facilities assign Code Team members who carry pagers or phones to receive alerts and allow response. Sometimes, Code Team members are alerted by an overhead speaker announcing "Code Blue, room___," but many hospitals avoid overhead announcements because they alarm patients and families.

Wherever the team comes from, it will always have a team leader, usually the physician, who is in charge. The team leader assesses the patient and the heart rhythms and orders the drugs and procedures needed. There is an algorithm of response pattern, called Advanced Cardiac Life Support (ACLS) that describes how to respond. The physician leader is not the only responder. It gets crowded during a code!

Code teams commonly also include someone to manage the airway (either anesthesiology or respiratory therapy) and advanced nurses (also trained in ACLS) to administer the drugs and hang the drips needed to control the cardiac rhythm and save the patient. In some facilities, a pharmacist responds and helps calculate the weight-based drugs needed, chaplains may provide spiritual support for families and staff and police officers may be present to help control hallways and clear elevators to take the patient to the intensive care unit (ICU) after a successful resuscitation. You may also see people from the laboratory coming to draw blood.

If the hospital is a teaching hospital (meaning it has contracts with schools for healthcare professionals), then various students will be present. In addition to all of those people, of course, family members are usually there. Most hospitals allow family members to be present if they are not being disruptive. Studies actually show that it is comforting to the family to see how very hard the team works to save their loved one. If a family member is present, nurses try to have one nurse or the chaplain assigned to help them by answering questions or interpreting events. This is another time when the nurse's tender loving care is needed.

After the Code

There are of course two possible outcomes to a code response: successful with the patient still alive or unsuccessful and the patient dies. Nursing tasks differ of course, depending on which outcome was achieved. In either case, the nurse who was recording the code will need to get a signature from the Team Leader after the code is over and before all the team members have dispersed.

After a successful code, the patient is transferred to the ICU where he or she can be watched carefully, since there is a higher risk for recurring abnormal heart rhythms immediately after a code. The nurse from the floor will accompany the team during this transfer and will report to the nurse in the ICU (see Chapter 5 about report). Nurses from the floor will also explain to the family and direct them to the ICU. And, of course, there is transfer paperwork to complete.

If the patient dies, the family will need support and comforting. Most facilities allow the body to remain in the room for a specific period of time to allow other family members to arrive and grieve. Take a look at the room before the family arrives and clean up as much as possible. After a code, there will be equipment and papers all over. There may be secretions, unsightly spills, or dirtied or bloodied linens depending on what procedures were attempted. Cleaning up those things, brushing the person's hair and smoothing the covers to create a more "normal" appearance is comforting to the family members when they arrive. Family mementos which may have been pushed out of the way during a code (such as pictures or balloons or cards) can be replaced on a clean table.

Different cultures respond to death in various ways, so find out what the family needs and try to provide as much support as possible. There is nothing wrong with crying with the family. Sometimes, the best comfort you can provide is to share their grief. It is not acceptable to break into uncontrolled sobs, though! The family needs you. So, empathize, sympathize and then provide the professional help they need. For instance, they may need practical advice about contacting a funeral home and making arrangements.

The chaplain or social service department of your hospital can be a helpful part of the team in assisting with arrangements. Most hospitals have morgues where bodies are taken if the funeral home does not come immediately. There is a specific procedure for preparing a body after death. Student nurses are not usually involved in this aspect of care.

Finally, take some moments to care for yourself if you have been involved in a code. In the immediacy of need, nurses tend to work automatically to do what needs to be done. Afterwards, there may be a let-down as hormones stop racing and the code completes. Naturally, if the patient has died, there is an added dimension of human compassion. We spend time getting close to our patients and families. It is a loss for us, too, when they die. Speaking to the chaplain, your instructor or other nurses and nursing students often helps handle the emotional response.

Example 8-1

Let's use the questions suggested in this chapter to consider what a student nurse might experience in a skilled nursing facility. It is not unusual for a student nurse to spend some days in a skilled facility to practice the basic nursing skills of bed baths, helping someone dress and feeding the dependant patient. Here's an example of what a student nurse log for a nursing home might look like:

- **Name of the unit/area/facility.** Magnolia Nursing Home
- **Purpose of the special area: why are patients sent there? Will the procedure or treatment be diagnostic or actually treat the patient's problem? If it is a treatment, will it cure the problem? If not, what problems may remain for the patient?** This is a resident facility for older people who can't take care of themselves anymore. We are helping these people get baths and feeding them. We don't really have any patient assigned to us, like we do when we're in the hospital. We just help whatever needs to be done on our hall. The patients are not actually having procedures; it's just a normal day for them. Oh, I forgot to call them residents. The nurse who talked to us when we first got there told us that the people live there. She said, "Remember that the residents don't live where we work. We work where they live." I thought about that for a minute and she's right. I thought it would be depressing going to a nursing home; but there are some nice people there. One old guy was telling me about the first time he saw a television! It was strange to think he didn't have one all along.
- **What type of healthcare workers staff the unit and what does each do for the patient? Especially focus on the nursing roles.** Most of the work is

done by the nursing aides. There was one nurse on each side, but I didn't really see her with the patients. The nurses stayed mostly in the nurse's station and checked the charts and when the aides would have a question or problem, the nurse would go see the patient. Sometimes, they called the doctor or spoke with the family. Medicines were given by a tech! I thought only nurses could give medicine, but the tech did it for everyone. The nursing aides took blood pressure, gave baths and helped the people who needed help getting dressed. We worked with the aides getting the people dressed and feeding them.

- **Is there any preparation required before the patient goes to the unit? Does a nurse assist this preparation? How?** No, because the patients live here, they're not really getting a procedure. Although, some of them go for therapy, crafts, or there is a bus that takes some out for trips.
- **What does the experience feel like to the patient?** I asked one of the ladies how she liked living here, and she said it was OK. Her daughter worked in a job where she traveled a lot, so she couldn't stay at her house any more. She missed her daughter; but liked having someone around all the time.
- **What will happen after the patient leaves the area? What are the nursing responsibilities, if any, afterwards?** Most of them don't leave; they live here. But there are a couple of people who came here after surgery and just aren't strong enough yet to go back home. Like one woman had a total hip replacement surgery; she will keep doing physical therapy until she is strong enough to go back to her own home.
- **Note any specific tasks you were able to perform for the patient while on the unit.** I helped one man use the shower. There is a big shower room. The guy sat on a rolling stool with a kind of donut seat (a hole in the middle) so we could spray up on his genital area while he was sitting down. I had never seen anything like that but it worked better than sponging him off in the bed. One of the other nursing students and I gave another patient—oops, resident—a bed bath and put new sheets on while the patient was in bed. It was just like we practiced in the lab, by rolling them from one side to the next. Then we helped them eat their lunch. It's harder than I thought to give someone a bite at a time. I mean, I didn't hardly know how much to put on the spoon at a time, or which thing they would like next!

Example 8-2

One of the specialty units students enjoy visiting is the ER. There are often opportunities to perform clinical skills, so look for them and let the staff know which ones you can perform (in other words, skills that you have completed in the lab at school and been told you can now do with a patient under supervision) so they call you when those skills are needed. You will likely have a chance to perform a phlebotomy (blood sample draw), possibly a urinary catheterization (to get a sterile sample checking for urinary tract infection), start an IV and maybe even perform CPR. Refer to skills performance as discussed earlier in this chapter.

Another learning opportunity in the ER is to perform focused assessments. When you are caring for a patient on the regular hospital floor, you will do a complete head-to-toe assessment. This allows you to check all patient systems and be sure you haven't missed anything. However, in the ER, staff focuses mainly on the system that is involved in the immediate problem. So pay attention to the assessment and diagnostic tests done for different patient problems and think through the reasons for them.

Here is a sample format for a simple log you might use to track what you did in the ER during your shift.

Clinical Log—Emergency Room

- **Skills performed and your comments:**

- **Assessments observed and comments:**

- **Diagnostic tests and what results showed:**

Example 8-3

Another special project you may do as part of clinicals might be a formal teaching project. This is more than simply instructing the patient and/or family during the clinical shift. In addition to that as part of regular nursing care, you might choose (or be assigned) a specific topic to teach and write up as a paper.

Here is a sample of a rubric that might be used to help you focus on each aspect of formal patient education.

TABLE 8-1   Patient Teaching Project

Student name _____ Date _____

Topic	Content	Possible Points	Points Earned
Client Assessment			
	Learning needs	10	
	Readiness/motivation to learn	5	
	Barriers to learning	5	
	Others to include in teaching/why	2	
Goals and Objectives (Planning)			
	Identify which learning need will be addressed and why	4	
	Goal and objectives for this teaching session	10	
	Prioritize other learning needs you won't have time to teach	4	
	Address how you might meet them in future shifts/ visits if this was your full time job	2	
Content (Implementation)			
	Specify what exactly you taught	20	
	Identify the realm of learning	2	
	Sources you used for content	2	
	Method of instruction	2	
	Describe the session	5	
	Patient information you provided	5	
	Documentation in chart	2	
Evaluation			
	Of client learning:		
	Effectiveness of session	5	
	Evidence goals/objectives were met	5	
	Explain if objectives not met and why	2	
	Of yourself as patient educator:		
	Identify positive aspects	4	
	How could you do better?	4	

Example 8-4   Doctor's Orders Project

Doctors orders legally define many aspects of our patients' care. The nurse needs to understand what it takes to follow up on orders. Please complete the following chart: the doctor's order at the top of the column is the first step and the order being carried out with the patient is the final step. What happens in between? Who is responsible for what? List each step, each action and indicate whose responsibility each step is. The charge nurse, staff nurses, unit secretary, policy and procedure manual, etc., can help you with this.

TABLE 8-2   From Doctor's Order to Nursing Action

Doctor writes order for medications or IV	Doctor writes order for consult	Doctor writes order for activity or diet	Doctor writes order for discharge
The patient receives the medications or IV	The consulting doctor visits the patient	The patient receives the diet or activity, etc.	The patient is discharged

Example 8-5   School Clinical Experience

Another specialty area you may be assigned is a public school. Student nurses may be sent to the schools to provide another pediatric experience. Below are guidelines you might use to understand the school-age child and the nurse's role in the schools.

Complete the assessment of:
- The school and student population (2 points): location, size, student population, socioeconomic level(s) of students

- Required health screens (6 points): immunizations, vision, hearing, scoliosis, nutrition needs, developmental stage(s)
- Types of special needs children (5 points): are there kids with developmental delays? Medical diagnosis? Medical equipment such as feeding tubes, wheelchairs, etc.? What is the nurse's role in their care? Who provides the special care? What are the classroom teachers taught?
- Structure of the clinic (5 points): physically describe or draw diagram/floor plan. Who works there? What level of nursing education? What about volunteers?
- Identify any barriers to care (2 points): money, language, culture, etc.
- Assessment of a child seen (10 points): you should assist with the care of children coming to the clinic. For one of them, write up an assessment: chief complaint, physical findings, pertinent history, needs, actions, etc.

Planning
- Describe laws affecting school care (5 points): do any of the Nurse Practice Acts address nursing in the schools? State laws about immunization, American with Disabilities Act, Board of Education regulations, etc. How do they affect the school nurse? Everything except medications in the school
- Rules regarding medications (5 points): medications are given in the school; what rules govern this practice?
- Protocols for care in school (3 points): are there policies/procedures/protocols? What types of care do they cover? If not, what areas do you think would be good to have protocols for and why?
- Prevention programs (4 points): are there programs in place designed to prevent health problems? Pregnancy? Smoking? Drugs? If so, describe them and the nurse's role if any. If not, what programs do you think would be beneficial?
- Define an Individual Education Plan (IEP) for a special needs child (2 points): how is the school nurse involved?

Interventions
- Cares given in the clinic (10 points): describe what you saw provided and/or what type of care can be provided if needed by the student. What is the nurse's role in each case?
- Teaching done (3 points): describe what you saw or what might be taught
- Medications (7 points): describe what you saw or what might be done. What procedures were followed? What is the nurse's role? What is the responsibility of student? Parent? Doctor?
- First Aid (3 points): describe what you saw or might see
- Referrals/teamwork (2 points): how does the nurse use other caregivers to meet the students' needs? Describe what you saw or what might be done.

Evaluation

- Of the setting (5 points): contrast health care in school setting versus hospital and with children versus adults. What was different about caring for students in the school? What was similar? What accommodations did you observe (or might need to be made) with the age of the child?
- Of yourself in this setting:
  - Personal reflections (2 points): what did you think about this experience?
  - Participation and meeting objectives (3 points): describe how you did or did not make use of this school experience and meet your objectives

Paper

- Spelling, grammar, punctuation, and format (5 points will be subtracted for errors or not following instructions, etc.)
- References (5 points): you must cite your references: where did you find the information used in the paper? If you quote something directly, it must be footnoted.

Chapter 9

Wrapping It Up—
Postconference

What Is It?

At the end of a clinical day, students will usually gather formally for an opportunity to discuss the day's experiences. This is referred to as postconference. Postconference can be viewed as a form of educational debriefing. This educational debriefing becomes another learning opportunity if it is embraced by the faculty and students.

In clinical education, postconference allows a time for sharing and expert input from the faculty facilitator to answer questions or direct further thought. It also provides the instructor with more insight into each student's level of understanding and experiences of the clinical day. Another advantage to postconference is to allow vicarious learning, as individual students reflect on experiences they had, thus turning them into learning experiences for the others. For the nursing student, postconference is a valuable time to show the instructor what has been accomplished and understood. It also provides the ability to learn through other students' experiences.

To get the most from postclinical conference, it helps to be an active participant. Being an active participant requires two components: (1) thinking and considering what you have experienced and then sharing freely, and (2) listening actively to the instructor's instructions and questions and to other student's comments. Use both of these approaches to make the most of postconference. Let's look at each aspect separately.

Sharing Tips—Thinking and Considering Before You Share

At the end of a clinical day, you are likely to be surprisingly tired. Eight or 12 hours of providing physical care for people, listening to their concerns, running the halls from nursing station to patient rooms and back again, lifting and supporting and all the while thinking hard can be exhausting! Once you finally sit down in the chair in postconference, it may wash over you just how tired you are.

The tendency for some is to sit back, take a breath and simply let the conversation take place around them without participating. Some students are tempted to rest, text, or tune out. Don't allow yourself to fall into these traps. Plan to make this an extension of your clinical learning because that is exactly what it is.

If you manage your time to allow a biological break before postconference, you can be ready. Refer to the time management discussion in Chapter 3. Please note that it is recommended that you begin leaving your patient about 30 minutes before postconference. This allows you to say goodbye to your patient and thank you to the staff nurse who worked with you. You can handle any final requests they have, assure your charting is complete and report off (refer to Chapter 5). And then you can get a drink, take a bathroom break and make it to postconference on time and ready to participate.

Follow the lead of your clinical instructor and respond to what is asked. Maybe you will be asked to share a clinical skill you performed or an example of patient assessment that was interesting. The instructor may want you to discuss what you saw of the role of the nurse during the shift or an example of a problem that you solved. Whatever the request, spend a minute or two thinking back over the shift.

Students often have trouble recounting examples of things they did well. We have been conditioned not to brag about ourselves. But your clinical instructor needs to hear these specific stories, both to evaluate your practice and also to direct you further and deeper. For instance, after completion of a skills performance, students tend to focus on aspects they missed or did not do well. Yet there are usually many things well done in the same skill, totally ignored by the student.

Think about what skills you were able to use during the shift so you can share them in postconference. Let's say you performed a sterile Foley catheterization on a male patient. Offer to share the experience by pointing out first what you did well. Did you: look up the Policy and Procedure of the hospital? Find all of the supplies with minimal help? Review the procedure in your mind before going into the patient's room? Explain to your patient? Wash your hands? All of these aspects of skills performance are vitally important and yet often not recognized by the student. Mention them! Celebrate them! And yes, brag about remembering each of these crucial and important steps.

Maybe your patient was worried about the procedure and you took time to listen to the fears and reassure the patient. Share how you did that. This is another example of nurses making a difference and your instructor and the other students need to hear it. Don't forget to include why the skill was needed: what information was it going to provide for diagnosis, or what patient problem was it going to help? With a sterile catheterization, for instance, the goal may be to get a specimen to identify a possible infection or it may be to leave a catheter in place because the person cannot void. Sharing your understanding of the value of the skill shows that you have clinical reasoning, which is helpful for your instructor to see.

Next, relate the actual skill performance itself. Your instructor may have been there or you may have received permission to perform the skill with your patient's staff nurse. Step-by-step, relate what you did so the other students can picture it and review. If there was something different about performing the skill for a real patient instead of in the lab, share that. For instance, maybe you were involved in the recovery room and had the opportunity to insert an airway. Choosing the correct size as you did in lab class is similar, but it is likely much easier to slide the airway in place on a real person with saliva than on the manikin in the lab! Sharing this practical aspect will reassure other students who perform it in the future.

If you relate tasks completed to something you learned in lecture, that is a bonus for you.

For instance, nursing students learn early in their training how to listen with a stethoscope to lung sounds. Most people do not have lung problems, and the normal sounds you hear are of air going in and out. So when you begin to identify lung sounds that are not normal and relate them to what you are studying in your lecture class, it really makes your learning more concrete and shows the instructor that you are putting it all together.

You may have heard something in the lungs that didn't sound "normal" but you weren't sure what it was. Have your clinical instructor or the staff nurse for the patient listen with you and identify it. Then think about why you are hearing this abnormal sound. Discuss possibilities in postconference. Relate it to the pathology and relate it to other aspects of your assessment (is the patient short of breath or coughing?). See how sharing your thoughts and possibilities allows instruction and discussion?

Actively participating in the sharing of postconference is quite valuable. Sometimes you will learn just as much through listening.

Active Listening is Vicarious Learning

Other students in your clinical group have been caring for their own patients, seeing different pathologies, experiencing other situations and working with different nurses.

Procedures: Aspects to consider and discuss in postconference
- Why was the procedure needed?
- What patient benefit is expected to come?
- Was there any patient preparation or anything the nurse needed to complete, before the procedure?
- What was the role of the nurse during the procedure?
- What did the procedure feel like to the patient?
- Was there any concern or special needs after the procedure was completed?

Figure 9-1   Procedures: aspects to consider and discuss in postconference.

As they share observations and stories, picture what they are describing. Ask questions; try to put what you hear into context. One student's story can turn into a valuable discussion when the other members of the clinical group get involved.

Sometimes, students have an opportunity to see something rare or participate in an interesting procedure. For instance, at times, a special type of intravenous line may be inserted by the doctor at the bedside (called a central line). Not every student may get an opportunity to observe this, so hearing a first hand report is the next best thing. Listen actively to the report and ask questions if you can't get a clear picture.

Both the student sharing and the students listening need to consider similar aspects of a reported procedure. Consider these aspects:

- **Why was the procedure needed?**
- **What benefit was expected for the patient?**
- **Was there any preparation of the patient or nurse before the procedure?**
- **What was it like for the patient to experience it?**
- **What was the role of the nurse during the procedure?**

Your discussion in postconference will be more helpful, and your instructor will be more impressed, when you listen and share in this manner.

Let's say you were in the emergency room during the shift and watched while the doctor inserted a chest tube. It is helpful to tell the other students what you saw and to answer their questions. However, how much more impressive would it be if you prepare a little beforehand and anticipate some of their questions as you share:

- **Why was the procedure needed?** The patient had been stabbed in the chest. He was in with respiratory distress. Rate was 38 and shallow; he was sweating, coughing blood and gasping. The pulse oximetry was only 90%, and his lips were kind of blue around the edges (this is called cyanosis).
- **What benefit was expected for the patient?** Obviously, this injury cut through the chest, ripped the pleural lining of the lungs and so all of the outside air and blood

had rushed in and collapsed the lung. It was dramatic—when you listened to his chest, you couldn't hear any breath sounds with your stethoscope on that side.

- **Was there any preparation of the patient or nurse before the procedure?** Everything happened fast. We had him sitting up straight so he could breathe easier and put oxygen on through a nasal cannula. The emergency room nurse got a chest tube tray and some sterile gloves. She told the patient that the doctor was going to put a tube in his side so his lung could open back up and he could breathe easier. He seemed scared. I held his hand.
- **What was it like for the patient to experience it?** Watching the doctor push that big tube in seemed rough. I mean they only gave him some pain medicine and then felt around on the ribs. Then a bit of local anesthetic and boom! The chest tube was pushed through! Immediately, you could see blood come out into the plastic chambers attached to the tube. What surprised me was that the patient seemed more relieved than hurt. That tube was big, but he just calmed down almost right away.
- **What was the role of the nurse during the procedure?** The nurse was awesome through the whole thing. You could see that just the way she talked to him, he felt safer. And even before the doctor asked for anything, she had it ready—like holding up the bottle of lidocaine so the doctor could fill the syringe and having the chamber ready to hook up the chest tube. She also let me see what was happening and got me right up close. Once the doctor heard her explaining things to me, they all started pointing out different stuff, like the suction and the drainage. Even when the x-ray people came, they showed me the film and you could really see where the lung was collapsed.

See how thinking through these questions before postconference allows you to share in a more thorough way? Your instructor will be pleased with the clinical reasoning you show

Example 9-1

It is first semester for a group of 10 students in their first clinical rotation. Postconference is scheduled for 1400–1500 in one of the hospital's conference rooms. The clinical instructor has indicated that today's goal for postconference is sharing a human interest story from each student's patient and discussing how it affects plans for nursing care.

Evaluate the following two postconference stories and plans.

1. One student nurse's story is that her patient was very nice and wanted to know all about the student's children. The student had a wonderful day sharing stories

of her kids and concluded that it showed her patient's loneliness. Her plan was to bring pictures the next day to share with the patient.

2. Another student shared that she had seen the staff nurse assigned to the patient, "make her get up and walk even though the patient didn't want to. After all she had surgery only yesterday and was really sore." The student nurse concluded that her nursing care plan would include respecting the patient's desire for rest and not forcing them to do things they don't want to.

Author's response: One good aspect of each of these students' responses is that they had listened to the instructor's request and had each shared a story that exemplified what was asked. This is one example of active participation in postconference and good listening. Each student gave a human interest story as asked and each student included an example of how it would impact their nursing care.

Regarding student 1: this student showed interaction with her patient. She obviously spoke with the patient and made an emotional contact with her patient. That aspect was good.

However, her story shows that the interaction featured herself and her child; not the patient. Remember in Chapter 1 when we discussed that our care needs to focus on the patient? As a professional nurse, you need to direct the conversation and utilize it to discover about your patient. It is all about them, not us. This student fell into the common mistake of making conversation about herself.

Students may argue: "But the patient asked me about myself, I was just being polite." Human nature and normal socialization train us to respond in this way. However, we can and should practice politely redirecting the conversation. For instance, when asked about our children, we could briefly respond honestly and then immediately redirect. You might say for instance, "I've been blessed with four children. I notice these pictures here on your window sill. Are these your children? Please tell me about them." See how this type of response, while still answering the question, allows the student to learn about the patient.

The value of redirecting conversations toward the patient is that we gather more information that may impact our plans. Whereas the student nurse in our example planned to bring pictures of her own children to show her patient, this would still have kept the focus on the student. We may discover that the patients' adult children live out of state and cannot help after discharge. Or we may learn that the patient's church is quite active in providing meals to shut-in parishioners. By keeping the conversation about the patient, we are respecting them as individuals and learning things that may help us provide better care.

Regarding student 2, who was offended that the patient's staff nurse "forced her to walk" so soon after surgery: as mentioned previously, the good thing is that the student did bring up a point that responds to the instructor's request. So that is good.

But the concern voiced indicates the students' inexperience. A good clinical instructor will use this type of situation to praise the student for empathizing with the patient.

The instructor would then explain why the staff nurse was encouraging activity and ambulation in this postoperative patient. Nursing students learn early in training what complications of immobility are. When a person is inactive, every body system is negatively impacted: skin sores can develop, clots in the leg are more likely, lung infections (pneumonia) can occur and the intestines slow down, causing constipation. These are only some of the possible consequences of a patient staying in bed. One of the most helpful, basic nursing interventions is to get your patients up and walking.

So the staff nurse was correct to encourage the patient to walk. What the student nurse needs to take away from this clinical experience is how important it is to explain clearly to patients why we are directing them to do specific things. Once patients understand how they gain from walking after surgery (or following a certain diet or taking medication, etc.), they are more likely to comply with the instruction. This is a big part of what an exceptional nurse can do for a patient in the clinical setting. Providing them with a clear understanding of how choices impact their health or recuperation empowers them to make good choices.

So, by actively sharing in postclinical conference, each student has provided a learning opportunity for themselves and the entire clinical group. What can other students in the group can take away from postconference? Through active listening to the previous stories, each student can learn and be ready to apply lessons learned in future clinical days. One lesson is to keep the focus on the patient and redirect a conversation. Other students actively listening to this postconference will also remember the importance of taking action to minimize complications of immobility. Another lesson is to explain why we are asking people to behave in certain ways.

Example 9-2   Sharing Mistakes

Let's consider another example:

Most clinical groups are small, 10 students for example, so the group cultivates a feeling of support for each other. Within that context, student nurses often use postconference to share "close calls" or actual mistakes that either happened to them or that they saw on their unit that clinical day. This benefits everyone if you are comfortable doing it.

For instance, one student nurse in her second semester was preparing to give an injection. She had done a perfect job of calculating how much drug to pull up from the multidose vial. She had properly discussed why the drug was ordered (how it would benefit the patient) and what anatomic landmarks to use for the site of the injection.

Those were the aspects of the injection she had been worried about, so when they were completed very well she felt such relief that, when she went to give the injection, she did not check the patient's name and medical record number again.

Checking the name and medical record number were first semester skills she had demonstrated previously but in this situation had forgotten to use. The instructor reminded her so she could correct the error before giving the injection. When she shared this in postconference, all of the other student nurses received an important reminder. Because she was willing to share, others may have been spared the same error.

Another student shared how her patient's mother almost led her to make a mistake. The student was caring for a patient who was 25 years old but had a previous head injury that left him physically and mentally impaired. After the student nurse helped him with morning care (cleaning up and shaving), she told his mother she would check if he could get up and sit in the chair. The mother assured her it was fine, "The physical therapist had him walking yesterday." But the student checked with the nursing staff and found out that he needed a special brace before getting up. If she had gone by what the mother told her, the patient might have fallen and possibly been injured. The student shared this and everyone was reminded to check orders and use staff member input as the final word.

You are not required in postconference to share errors, but the benefit to the group of doing so is clear. In fact, some students are afraid their instructor will grade them lower for the admission, but a good clinical instructor will applaud students' sharing close calls and errors as representative of the students' professionalism.

Example 9-3

The flip side to sharing errors is sharing triumphs!

There are times when your clinical assignment becomes something different than first expected. The student nurse was in her first semester and her patient was nonresponsive. Cancer had spread through her body, and between the disease and the narcotic pain control she required total care. So the student expected to bathe her and change her sheets, clean her mouth, and provide other basic care. Indeed this was what happened until lunchtime of the second day when the patient's breathing became erratic. First, she would breathe shallow and very slowly. Then the student reported she gasped, sucking in a deep breath quite loudly. Then there was no breath for a number of seconds. When the instructor came in answer to the student's page, it was clear that the patient was now close to death and the breathing pattern (called Cheyne-Stokes) was a sign that death may come soon. Since the patient had an order in place that there was to be no resuscitation (DNR 5 do not resuscitate) when she died, the nursing goal became comfort and emotional/spiritual support for the patient and family.

The student was given the choice of continuing to care for the patient (with the help of the nursing staff) or taking a different assignment, since end-of-life care had not been covered yet at school. However, the student now had two shifts with the patient and felt close to the adult daughter, so she opted to stay. The instructor gave her quick instruction on how to support the family and patient. The patient died within 1 hour.

In postconference, the student shared the experience and helped all of the students consider how they would assist a patient and family when the time came. Discussion not only covered the physical signs of impending death, but also the emotional aspects for family and for the student. Nursing not only starts from the heart. It also ends from the heart. The student experienced that and shared the compassion and privilege it is to help someone die comfortably and with dignity and support.

The student nurse shared the daughter's comments after her mother's death: "Thank you for being there with us. I know you helped mom—and you sure helped me." There was not a dry eye in postconference that day. Nursing students enter the profession with the idea of helping patients. This was a clear demonstration of just how valuable nurses can be.

Example 9-4   Sharing Clinical Opportunities

It is not unusual for nursing programs to provide assignments to departments where the student will be an "observer" (see Chapter 8). When you have visited a hospital department or community facility, postconference is a perfect opportunity to share the experience with other students who will be going there, too, sometime during their clinical semester. Your feedback can set the stage for a better experience for them, and also let the clinical instructor know about the relative value of the experience for students.

For instance, one of the departments student nurses may spend a clinical day is in day surgery or the cardiac catheterization lab (cath. lab) to get opportunities to start intravenous lines. In postconference, it is helpful if students share hints learned: nurses who were especially helpful when you were there, patient situations encountered and how they were handled, how to position yourself for the best learning opportunity, etc.

If the observation day was outside of the hospital, there may be hints about finding the facility, parking, whether a refrigerator is available for lunch or other practical matters are invaluable. Another aspect to share with the instructor in postconference is whether the objectives could be met or not in the outside clinical experience. For instance, if the student nurse is sent to a pediatric clinic, one of the objectives may be to perform a physical assessment for children. If clinic personnel do not allow you to actually interact with the children and instead ask you to "watch," your instructor and the other students need to know that.

Example 9-5   Other General Tips and Examples for Postconference

- Arrive on time. Student nurses who are consistently late for postconference give the message that they do not have time management skills.
- Share in postconference any skills that you were able to perform with your staff nurse. Nursing instructors have many students in the hospital each clinical day and therefore are not present to personally observe everything. If your instructor allows you to perform a skill with other nurses supervising, be sure to share specifics of the opportunity. For instance, you might have done an insulin injection with your instructor before, so she tells you to do the next one with the staff nurse assigned to that patient. In postconference, share the results. Be specific: "my patient's blood sugar was 250, so we gave her two units of regular insulin according to the sliding scale order. I had the nurse show me where the insulin was kept in the medication room, but I drew it up myself as she watched; she watched me give it. The patient wanted me to use the arm since she always gives it to herself on the belly when she is at home." Being specific like this in your reports allows your instructor to have clear information about where you stand in your clinical progress.
- Another tip: ask questions. You are going to see patients with diagnoses you haven't yet studied. Ask about the pathologies and nursing cares for them. But think first before questioning. What system is affected by the disease? What is the usual function of the system and, therefore, what trouble might your patient have if that function is impaired? What might you expect to find on patient assessment because of the system compromise? Thoughtful questions are much appreciated and demonstrate to your clinical instructor that you are thinking. They also show the instructor how to help you get to the next level of understanding.

For instance, let's say you took care of someone who had a total knee replacement. You probably don't understand the specifics of the surgery, but you know the knee is supposed to bend to allow motor function. Therefore, walking and sitting are likely affected. State your understanding of this. But maybe your patient has a drain in the knee, or a cuff attached to a cooler-like contraption, or a clear plastic container and some mention of "auto-transfusion." Ask about these specific things within the context of what you do know. Again, this allows your instructor to gauge progress and help direct you to advance. Also, the discussion and explanations that follow your question will benefit the entire group.

Example 9-6   Another Postconference Plan for the New Student Nurse

---

Here is a suggestion for one or two post-conferences when you are new to clinicals: Have each student nurse give report on one patient using the format discussed in this book or the format preferred by your clinical instructor. All other students listen and take notes. Learning to take report is an important skill, too. After one student has given report to the group, discuss the report. Answer these questions: What were *good* aspects of the report that was given? Was there information missing? What medical terminology was used appropriately? What medical terminology could have been used instead of layman's terms? What could be improved in the overall report? What patient problems are identified in the report? Which are of the highest priority? Why? What actions could the nurse take to improve the patient's status?

Indeed, postclinical conference is an opportunity for vicarious learning—take advantage of it! Enjoy your patients and fellow students along the way. Remember—our patients are what nursing is all about and sharing the learning experiences advances all of us.

Chapter 10

Simulation—An Alternate Clinical Experience

WITH KELLY VANDENBERG, PHD, RN

*"My gosh! The first time I went into that lab, it was weird.
There were lots of hospital beds and for a minute I thought REAL
people were in them. Then I saw it was a bunch of dummies!"*

*"My instructor says we just can't get the space for as many clinical
days as the school needs. So we are going to use the simulation lab.
That just doesn't seem right! How can we be expected to take care
of real patients when we have to practice on manikins?"*

*"At first I wasn't sure about working in the simulation lab. I mean,
it seemed weird talking to a dummy with a camera rolling!
But actually we really got into it and afterwards it was cool to
watch the video."*

A book preparing you for clinical success would not be complete without a chapter on simulation. Nursing schools around the country are increasingly using simulation experiences either as preparation for clinical rotations or as a portion of the clinical experience. Many factors are driving this trend toward simulation: improved technologies that allow more realistic and interactive simulations, the demand from hospitals to prepare graduate nurses at a higher level and the nursing shortage pressuring colleges to increase class size with its resultant battle for clinical sites to provide experience for the students. Another factor pushing nursing schools into simulation is the ability to create a specific patient problem instead of waiting until the student actually sees it in the hospital. Enter technology to the rescue: simulated clinical experiences!

As a student nurse, you will likely encounter many training approaches to simulate real life clinical situations. Nursing schools have used simulation to help students learn for years. Time tested methods of simulation include students pretending to be the patient and practicing with each other or using an orange when practicing your first injection instead of a real patient. These simple scenarios are simulations of the low-tech kind. Improved technologies allow far more complex simulated experiences. This chapter will explore simulation as an alternate clinical experience.

Make It Real

As with all learning experiences, you have the power to make it count or to minimize it.

The key to turning a simulated clinical experience into a learning experience that is comparable to taking care of real patients is to approach it with that intent. Pretend this is a real patient. Any level of simulation will be valuable to you if you transfer in your mind this "pretend" patient into a real one. Act as if the patient is right there in the words that you speak, the actions you take and the responses you give.

How do you make it real? Here are some suggestions:

- Wear your student nurse uniform—when you dress the part, you more realistically play the part and that transfers to a more valuable learning experience.
- Carry your usual clinical equipment: stethoscope, watch with a second hand, bandage scissors, etc., whatever you are required to have for clinical shifts in the hospital.
- Talk during the simulation experience as if you were with a real patient. Even if your best friend is your pretend patient or the patient is a manikin who definitely does not look real, speak to them as if you were talking to the patient. Name the patient!
- Take advantage of the "role" you are assigned during the simulation. Get into it! You may be the patient, nurse, family member or some other role. Each role

allows you to empathize in a different way. One of the challenges of nursing is to appreciate the way your patient and their family members feel. The simulation experience is an opportunity to act out those feelings, which prepares you to better understand real patients. Become a terrific actor during simulated clinical experiences.

- Associate with other students who are open and participatory with these alternate simulation experiences. Attending the clinical simulation with those who are also open to treating the simulation experience as a real clinical experience elevates your opportunity to learn. Attending with students who treat it as a joke and laugh throughout will detract from your learning.
- Practice relaxation or anxiety-reducing techniques if you have performance anxiety triggered by these pretend patient situations.
- Take advantage of any extra practice time (sometimes called "open lab") offered to you as a student. The more familiar you become with the equipment and setting, the more practiced you become with the manikins, the better you will be able to allow yourself to let go and make it real!
- Prepare for the simulation experience. You will prepare for clinical experiences, too. Preparation may involve looking up a disease process, refining patient assessment techniques or planning the types of nursing interventions a particular patient may need. You may be invited to visit the manufacturer's Web site for an advanced preview of what to expect from the manikin your school uses.

Add the dimension of actually thinking about what you are doing, and you have deepened your learning and level of preparation. For instance, if you are simulating how to complete a bed bath, you could ask a series of questions about the patient: what is the medical reason the patient needs a bed bath instead of getting into the tub or shower? Are there aspects of the bath the patient could perform themselves, even though they can't get out of bed? If so, should you as their nurse encourage them to do those parts themselves? Why or why not? How does the patient feel during the bed bath? What can the nurse do to make this highly personal and potentially embarrassing task more comfortable?

All levels of simulation experience will be driven by their objectives. Just as your clinical experiences seek a specific type of patient who meets your clinical objectives, it is also important in your simulated clinical experiences to match the objectives of the simulation to the level of the student and the individual unit of study. It helps the student get the most out of the simulation if the objectives are clearly understood. Remember, the equipment and the computer software are simply tools to help you take care of patients.

Higher levels of simulation allow more complex thought, as the computer software and hardware show response to your actions. Evaluating the "patient" situation, your actions and the results of what you did is a wonderful way of learning. In fact, it is the

Category	Description	Examples
LOW	An educational environment used to train a student for a skill or patient situation.	Fellow students or family members role playing patient situations Practicing body mechanics as one student mimics the limitations of a cerebrovascular accident (CVA) and another assists with transfer or use of equipment Pretending to give a subcutaneous or intramuscular injection using an orange or piece of silicone material Using a hot dog to practice creating intradermal wheels for TB injection
MEDIUM	An educational environment that uses simple models or basic computer software to train nursing students for a skill or patient situation.	Checking blood pressure (BP) accuracy using an arm model with a small computer inside which can be programmed to specific BP readings Inserting a virtual IV through use of a computer program and attached hardware Catheterizing a simple model of the genitalia, without full body attached; or using squares of silicone with fake wounds to practice dressing changes Charting on an Electronic Health Record, a computer mock-up of a patient chart Preparing medications for administration using a Computerized Medication Cart Using manikins to practice and pass a cardiopulmonary resuscitation (CPR) course Using virtual software: programs that allow the student to manipulate the environment to care for a patient (resulting in a step by step analysis of what the student did right and what the student did wrong)
HIGH FIDELITY	An educational environment using a sophisticated, computerized human simulator manikin to allow students to practice patient scenarios and see the response of their interactions on the manikin (patient).	Utilizing full body manikins with computer insides and mechanisms that show changes in vital signs, cardiac rhythm, lung sounds, and heart sounds, and bowel sounds. They have more realistic skin and appearance and many blink their eyes. The chest may rise and fall with respirations. Some high fidelity simulators have simulated speech, as another person can "speak" through them. Training for advanced cardiac life support (ACLS) often occurs on a high fidelity human simulator. Using high fidelity equipment commonly involves multiple students; and makes interdisciplinary patient scenarios possible, i.e. including students in other health professions such as Respiratory Therapy, Physical Therapy, etc.
LIVE MODEL/ STAN- DARDIZED PATIENT	An educational environment that uses paid or unpaid actors to simulate a patient situation	Models: A person with an existing condition that may help students learn (example: a pregnant model for a woman's health course) Standardized Patients: Real people who volunteer to be trained on a specific condition or disease process. Medical schools commonly use standardized patients.

Figure 10-1

entire purpose of clinical experience. When you approach simulated clinical with all of this in mind, it really counts for clinical learning, no matter what level of simulation is used.

The chart on the previous page describes some types of simulation you may encounter at nursing school which may supplement or substitute for an actual clinical experience. The chart gives some examples but is not a complete listing of available resources. Since these new high fidelity technologies are recent and costly, your school may not use all types.

Low-Tech and Medium-Tech Simulation

Most simulations of the low-tech or medium-tech categories are used primarily to practice specific skills, as opposed to clinical substitutes. They are valuable for allowing repetition and assuring the steps of a procedure are mastered. A student can stick a plastic arm multiple times to practice starting an intravenous (IV) line or insert a tube through a fake nose and into the fake stomach to assure proper procedure is followed. When these individual tasks are discussed in relation to patient situations, they become more clinical and less a simple task.

A good clinical instructor will assist the student nurse to relate the task to a real patient situation before a skill performance in a simulation or in the clinical setting. The steps of the skill will be reviewed and mimicked, and the patient situation regarding the need for the skill will be discussed. You will be encouraged to think about potential risks, benefits and outcomes of the procedure in context of the patient. If your instructor does not incorporate the thought processes behind the skill, make this something you ask about or discuss with your fellow students.

Beyond these low- and medium-tech simulations, though, even more complex simulations have been developed. Recent technology has allowed nursing schools to use more realistic and involved simulation environments. The remainder of the chapter will focus on the latest technologies for high-fidelity simulations that use a patient simulator (manikin). These are the types of simulation experiences that most likely will substitute for a clinical shift.

High-Fidelity Simulation

Each high-fidelity simulation will involve a scenario. A scenario is like a plot in a movie. The scenario mimics situations you may encounter in your nursing career. The patient presents with a problem (it wouldn't be any fun if there wasn't a problem!). The nurse must fully assess and then take actions to help or resolve the problem. Family members or other healthcare providers may be part of the scene. Each actor/student is provided a script which sketches out basic roles. You may be provided with preparation materials to help you get ready for the scenario.

You attend the simulation and, after the nurse takes action, the patient status is made to change. If the nurse took appropriate action, the patient improves. Improper nursing intervention creates more problems for the patient. These patient responses are reflected in changes in vital signs or chest sounds or in patient verbalizations (through the "voice" of the instructor speaking through the manikin). This is the same thing that would happen in a hospital during a clinical shift.

After the simulation scenario has played out (it may take anywhere from a 10–60 minutes), there will be a discussion about it. This process is called debriefing and is extremely valuable. During debriefing, each student who played a role will discuss what happened in the simulation. The patient's problem, nursing interventions and patient responses will be reviewed. You have the opportunity to assess how well you did or what could be improved. There is quite a parallel here with the actual clinical experience.

For example, clinical shifts involve preparation, performing during the shift and then attending postconference to discuss the day's care. In most high-fidelity simulations, your instructor will provide you with assignments to prepare, you will provide care to the human simulator and conclude with a review called debriefing. High-fidelity simulations can be approached as another clinical "site" that requires preparation, care and debriefing. Let's look at each aspect of the process individually and consider how you can create the best experience for yourself.

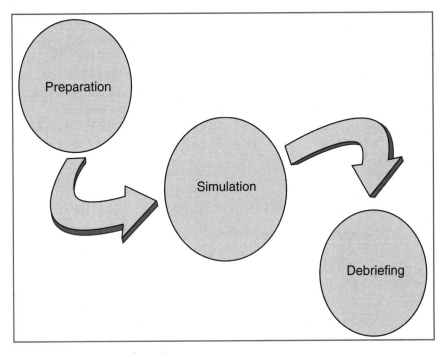

Figure 10-2   Process of simulation.

Student Preparation

Preparation is critical to your high-fidelity experience just as preparation is critical to your clinical site visit. If you avoid these assignments you limit the learning experience. For high-fidelity simulations, some additional information or material may be included depending on your program. Some nursing programs have developed videos or orientations that will allow you to see the human patient simulator and describe the environment in which you will be working. In addition, some companies that make the simulators have Web sites that provide a view and description of the capabilities of their human simulators. Although the intent is to create an environment close to reality, recognizing the differences between simulated manikins and real people will help you.

- The appearance of the manikin will be the first difference you encounter. Although these wonderful computer-generated programs can simulate a disease process, they are far from real. The plastic skin and limited facial and body movements may startle you at first. It is important that you do not let this flaw prevent you from practicing your nursing skills. Make a choice to treat this manikin as a patient. Treat the human simulator as you would a real patient.
- Understand the manikins may have makeup or props to support the scenario. Moulage is the term that refers to this preparation of the simulator. For example, let's say the scenario describes a 67-year-old African American female who presents to the emergency room via ambulance after a motor vehicle accident. Your human simulator may have on a wig, clothes, and breasts to simulate a female, make up to simulate ethnicity, blood and lacerations to simulate injuries, and dressings, IVs, and IV pumps with fluids begun at the scene.
- Simulators come in a variety of sizes. Some manikins are large and bulky, some are small children or infants and there are even pregnant females! This is a great time to practice body mechanics when transferring a patient. Use the appropriate number of people to help transfer, and don't forget to put the bed or stretcher at a proper height.
- Functions of the human simulator vary:
  - Your human simulator may speak to you! Many students find the communication between the nurse and the simulator eerie at first, but soon become accustom to the interaction. Your human simulator's voice may be another student, instructor or staff member who has been given a script to follow as you care for your patient. This is a great way to practice your communication techniques. It is also a great way to collect information for your history and physical assessment. Remember, this is your patient!
  - Your human simulator has pulses (from neck to feet) that can be palpated. Depending on your scenario, these pulses may be strong, weak, or absent.

○ Your human simulator has heart sounds. The heart rate and types of heart sounds can be manipulated with the computer controls. You will be able to hear these heart sounds with your stethoscope. The heart sounds may sound mechanical with older models of human simulators, but great progress has been made in the newer models. Many simulations include a monitor that will provide you with additional data such as blood pressure, heart rate, oxygen saturation, electrocardiogram (EKG), etc.

○ Your human simulator has lung sounds! You will be able to use your stethoscope to hear lung sounds. Lung sounds can include crackles, wheezing or absent sounds, etc. This is a good time to practice your assessment skills. Make sure to listen to all lung fields. Older models of human simulators will not have posterior (back) lung sounds, but they all have anterior (front) lung sounds. Some recent human simulators have both posterior and anterior lung sounds. Again, finding out what type or model of human simulator your nursing program uses will help you understand the limitations.

○ Your human simulator has bowel sounds! You will be able to assess the bowel sounds (hyper, hypo or absent) by using your stethoscope.

○ Other functions that your human simulator may be capable of is the insertions of IVs, Foley catheters, central lines, intubation, nasal gastric tubes, ventilators, oxygen, suctioning, chest tubes, central lines and many more.

Simulation

If your nursing program provides you with high-fidelity simulations, you are the beginning of a new generation of nurses who have the opportunity to practice on manikins first instead of "real patients." You not only have the ability to learn from the experience, but you have the ability to learn from your mistakes without harm to a person. Many nurses from earlier generations are in awe of this opportunity you have!

After you have prepared for your scenario (plot) in your high-fidelity simulation and reviewed the functions of your human simulator, you will be ready to enter the simulation environment. Please note that each nursing program will have different equipment and various setups (individual rooms or one large room with different types and numbers of manikins).

Regardless of the type of room or equipment, your first encounter in this environment may be intimidating. You may be anxious because of the high-tech environment or the fact that you may be the lead nurse in charge. There will be faculty and instructors monitoring your progress, and usually video cameras are taping to be used during debriefing. It is important that you mentally prepare for this experience. Talk to other students who have used the simulation lab and get a clear picture of what to expect.

Although everyone's experience is unique, the more prepared you are, the more you can take advantage of the situation.

When you arrive for your high-fidelity simulation, your instructor will usually state the objectives for the simulation. A brief overview and orientation to the environment usually occurs. Most high-fidelity simulations involve a group or team of nursing students. You may be a part of a group of 2–8 students participating in the high-fidelity simulation. Student nursing roles may include lead nurse, assessment nurse, medication nurse, skills nurse, documentation nurse, etc. Other roles may include the patient's voice, a family member role, another healthcare worker or students assigned as observers of the scenario.

If you are assigned one of the nursing roles during simulation, you will be assessing the patient (the human simulator manikin) and taking actions to help whatever problem the patient is experiencing. If you are assigned one of the other supportive roles in the scenario, you will be given a script that describes what the problem is and suggests how you might play the role. Other students may be assigned to observe the scenario play out and look for certain actions by the nurse.

Your nursing school may also have the ability to provide simulations with team members from other disciplines, such as medical students, physical therapy students, respiratory therapy student or emergency medical service students. You may also encounter high-fidelity simulations with graduate and undergraduate students or students from different semesters. This is a wonderful time to develop communication skills, teamwork and to learn more about what other members on the healthcare team can do. Group involvement also brings multiple ideas and interactions from which you can learn.

If your high-fidelity simulation is being taped, your nursing program may have you sign a consent form that describes how the video will be used to enhance your learning experience. Some schools destroy or erase the videos after each use, while others may keep copies for educational purposes or individual student portfolios. You may want to ask your instructor what the video will be used for. Decisions are usually based on the costs of audio-visual systems, costs of storing large amounts of data, cost of media to record data, student access and confidentiality issues.

The video may actually be linked to the human simulator! These specialized video capabilities allow viewing the video, data from the monitor, interventions and documentation during the simulation. This type of camera is usually small and mounted in an area around your simulated environment. Some nursing programs record from a control room outside of your simulated environment. In that case, cameras are located on the ceiling and/or the head of the bed. There may simply be a regular video camera on a tripod. Although not all high-fidelity simulations use video in the debriefing portion of the process, the video does offer an objective point of view and additional means for the student to discover learning opportunities.

How do you feel about being videotaped?! For some, it sounds like fun and others feel anxiety about it. To help decrease anxiety, you may want to tape yourself while you practice other tasks and assessment skills. Reviewing the tape will help you discover ways to improve your skills and develop a comfort level of the "third eye" (camera, instructor, patient or family member). Other students develop an attitude of ignoring the camera during taping. Whichever makes you comfortable is fine.

In addition to the human simulator manikin and taping equipment, there are many other technologies, equipment and supplies present to act out the scenario. Most high-fidelity simulations will have a variety of technologies and supplies:

- Patient chart (paper chart or an electronic health record)
- Documentation (white board, paper or electronic health record)
- Phone or alert system to notify physician or crisis team of patient changes
- Bed or stretcher that will adjust heights or elevation of head of bed
- Monitor that can display multiple types of patient data such as EKG, heart rate, oxygen saturation, etc.
- Medication cart (with or without computerized medication administration records)
- Resources to investigate medications, disease processes, policies and procedures (either in book form or software on bedside computer or personal digital assistant)
- Supply cart with a variety of supplies
- Oxygen and oxygen tubing, suction, Foley catheters, IVs, IV pumps, feeding pumps, patient-controlled anesthesia (PCA), chest tubes, central lines, ventilators, etc
- Use your imagination about future technologies that will be developed!

Outside your environment, you may see microphones used for the patient voice, video camera (wall, ceiling or tripod) and computer stations used to view video during debriefing (in the same room, in an adjacent debriefing room or a classroom). Your instructor may be monitoring the high-fidelity simulation from the bedside or in a control room outside of the simulation environment. You may also see support staff adjacent to your simulated environment to assure that the equipment is operating properly.

Your human simulator will respond to your interventions. Remember to complete ongoing assessments as the scenario unfolds. Just as in actual clinical situations, the patient's original status changes with our interventions. Reassess and monitor your patient continuously. The findings of reassessment will determine additional needs and interventions.

Here is a simple scenario a beginning student might see in simulation:

The plot is that you are a staff nurse on a medical-surgical floor. One of your patients had abdominal surgery yesterday (nurses would say "the patient is 1 day post-op").

He has the original dressing on the abdomen, is receiving IV fluids and gives himself narcotic pain medication through his IV by pushing a little button (PCA). His wife is at the bedside reading a book when you enter.

You are the nurse. Another student is assigned to be the patient's wife. The human simulator in bed is the patient. There is an IV bag hanging, a pump labeled morphine PCA, and an abdominal dressing with a blood stain about half-dollar size. A portable machine is near the bedside; it takes blood pressure and pulse measurements. There is a camera on a tripod at the end of the bed recording the session.

Two students are watching from the side of the room. You can't see the instructor, but have been told she is behind a control desk. According to the script, you saw the patient an hour ago and he was stable; you are simply coming in the room to check up on him again. The "wife" had been given a script to suggest what kind of comments she should make during the simulation (but you don't know what her instructions are).

That is the set-up. Can you picture that? Let's follow it through.

You (the nurse): Knock on the door and say, "It's the nurse."

Wife, in a quiet voice: "Come on in, he's resting so peacefully, sshhhhhh."

You: "I'm glad he's comfortable. I just wanted to check in and be sure he's fine." You turn to the patient and note his eyes are closed, and he appears to be sleeping. You pull the covers back to check his dressing and notice there is no further bleeding. His color is pale.

Wife, interrupting your assessment, says, "Can't you wait on that? Just let him sleep? He was so restless earlier and I finally got him comfortable." There are many different responses students may make in this situation. . .

You, in a whisper, answer (possible response #1): "OK Mrs. Jones. I'll come back later. How long do you think he needs to rest?" *or*

You in a quiet voice, answer (possible response #2): "I will check quickly and quietly, but I need to be sure he's OK," and then you continue your assessment. You note his blood pressure is within his normal range, the pulse is slower than usual and he is breathing 14 times per minute. Since the blood pressure is fine and there is no further bleeding, you smile at the wife and quietly leave the room to chart that everything is fine. *or*

You, in a quiet voice, answer (possible response #3): "I will check quickly and quietly, but I need to be sure he's OK," and then you continue your assessment. You note his blood pressure is within his normal range, the pulse is slower than usual and he is breathing 14 times per minute. Since the breathing rate is slow, you attach a pulse oximeter, a small clip on the finger attached to a little box that measures oxygenation. While it is reading, you check the PCA pump to see how much morphine he has received because you know one of the effects of narcotic pain medicine is to suppress breathing. As you check the PCA pump, the wife asks: "What are you doing?"

You: "I just want to be sure he is not getting too much pain medicine, so I'm looking at the history." The patient continues to sleep as you and the wife talk.

Wife, sounding defensive: "What do you mean *too much* medicine? I thought that thing controlled it so he only got the right amount."

You: "There are limits programmed in. But it is just a machine; we check often to make sure the amount controls the pain without too much sedation. Another protection is that, if it is more than he needs for pain control, he will get sleepy and stop pushing his button. This keeps him from getting too much. Unless someone else pushes the button. Mrs. Jones, did you push the PCA button?" The scenario would continue.

See how each possible nurse response is different and allows you to practice how you would respond? And with each different nurse response, the patient's condition (through the control of the instructor at the controls) would change. For the nurses who left the room in possible response #1 and #2, the respiratory status would continue to worsen. The instructor may send the nurse back in the room and create an even more depressed respiratory status and lower oxygen rate. The blood pressure would fall and the pulse may get fast trying to compensate. If the nurse properly assessed this when returning to the room, she might administer oxygen, give Narcan (a medicine to reverse the effect of the narcotic) and call the doctor. If these steps were not taken, the patient status might continue to deteriorate until he was not breathing at all (this is called respiratory arrest)!

For possible response #3, if the pulse oximeter reading was good and the wife stopped pushing the button for her husband, the patient (human simulator) would awaken and all would be fine.

See how flexible the simulation is? It literally unfolds as you go, depending on your assessments and interventions for the patient. You are learning how to respond in an environment where no one is really harmed. The specific situation of respiratory suppression from narcotic administration can be created without waiting for it to actually happen to a real patient.

It might surprise you that during the simulation you may develop caring feelings toward the human simulator (just as you would for a real patient). Many instructors have found that it is more useful to stop the simulated environment before the human simulator dies because of the emotional response of students. The emotional response overshadows the purpose or objectives planned for the simulated environment. Stopping the high-fidelity simulation and discussing mistakes provides a window of opportunity for teaching, reinforcement of skills and critical thinking. Of course, there are scenarios that have objectives related to end-of-life issues where the human simulator dies as part of the scenario.

Debriefing

After you have completed your simulation, you may hear "cut," "that's a wrap," "congratulations you have completed your simulation" or maybe "your simulation is now complete." Regardless of how your instructor ends the session, you will most likely feel a sense of relief. Congratulations! You have experienced your first simulation! But it is not complete until the debriefing is finished.

Some feel the debriefing process impacts learning even more than the simulation itself. The debriefing process is a structured environment to help you discover what went right or wrong, what could have been done better, etc. Go into debriefing with an open mind and engage in the conversations—you will benefit tremendously. Although the scrutiny of debriefing may seem intimidating, it is tremendously helpful. Avoid being defensive so you can learn! During the debriefing process, you will learn from your fellow team members, your instructor and most of all, yourself!

There are a variety of ways your instructor will lead you through the debriefing process. Some plan a small break so you can regroup. During this time, you may have exciting conversations as you discuss the high-fidelity simulation with fellow team members. Some instructors (depending on the time constraints) will go straight into the debriefing. The first question usually is, *"how did you feel about the simulation?"* Many comments, feelings and ideas will be shared as you discuss the simulation. Engaging in this emotional dump can be therapeutic! Then, you will focus on the objectives of the simulation.

The instructor may have a list (on paper or in their minds) of what they wanted you to accomplish during the process. During debriefing, all team members will consider how these aspects of the scenario were met. Actively considering what went on is important. It's also important to recognize what you did well! Students often have trouble noting their abilities and tend to focus on what was missed: "I forgot to wash my hands" (or some other step in a procedure). Yet, there were likely many other aspects that you did well. Part of being a professional is recognizing what you did well so it can be repeated.

If the simulation was videotaped, you may become critical of how you looked (I don't like my hair up in that clip) or some other aspect of the video (does my voice really sound that high?!) that isn't really as important as the actions you took. Try to focus on what actions were taken and the quality of your interactions and assessments instead.

Debriefing becomes a self-reflection exercise in recognizing both the positive aspects of the simulation and the parts that could be improved. What aspects of the simulation are considered during debriefing? The debriefing focuses on the patient's problem and how you, as the nurse, responded to the problem. Your level in nursing school is considered, as new students are not expected to show the mastery of a student who is about to graduate. Here are some questions that may be asked:

- What was the patient's problem?
- Was the assessment correct for the problem? What aspects of assessment were done well? What aspects could have been improved? Was the nurse able to identify the patient's problem?

- What nursing interventions were taken for the problem? Were they proper? Were they timely?
- What information was gained from the supporting roles? Was it realistic?
- Did the patient's condition change during the simulation? Why? Did the nurse recognize the change? Why or why not?
- Were other interventions taken in response to the change in the patient's condition? What aspects were proper; and what might have been done differently?

Let's take those debriefing points and explore them for the simulation example we discussed earlier. The plot of the simulation is that you are a staff nurse on a medical-surgical floor. Your patient is 1 day postoperative after abdominal surgery. He has the original dressing on, is receiving IV fluids and gives himself narcotic pain medication through his IV (PCA). His wife is at the bedside reading a book when you enter.

First, debriefing on possible responses #1 and #2:

- What was the patient's problem? *Respiratory suppression from too much narcotic.*
- Was the assessment correct for the problem? *No.* What aspects of assessment were done well? *The nurse was sensitive to the wife's concern for patient rest.* What aspects could have been improved? *No assessment was done in the first example; the nurse let the patient's wife dictate her nursing care. In example #2, minimal postoperative assessment was done of the dressing and vital signs, but the low respirations were not recognized.* Was the nurse able to identify the patient's problem? *No, because the assessment was not done.*
- What nursing interventions were taken for the problem? Were they proper? Were they timely? *The nurse left the room. No interventions for respiration were taken.*
- What information was gained from the supporting roles? *The wife's part was played well, we learned the patient was resting and she did not want him disturbed.* Was it realistic? *Very realistic.*
- Did the patient's condition change during the simulation? Why? Did the nurse recognize the change? Why or why not? *If the example had continued, we would have seen deterioration in the respiratory status.*
- Were other interventions taken in response to the change in the patient's condition? What aspects were proper; and what might have been done differently? *(Not followed up in the example.)*

Let's answer the same debriefing questions for possible response #3:

- What was the patient's problem? *Respiratory suppression from too much narcotic.*

- Was the assessment correct for the problem? *Yes.* What aspects of assessment were done well? *Pulse oximeter and checking the PCA pump history readings. The student nurse also did a good job of assessing if the wife was pushing the PCA button.* What aspects could have been improved? *It would have been good to listen to the chest with a stethoscope and also to awaken the patient and assess for his level of consciousness: did he know his own name and where he was? Could he respond to voice commands? Could he move his extremities? This is another indicator of the degree of sedation.* Was the nurse able to identify the patient's problem? *Yes.*

- What nursing interventions were taken for the problem? *The student nurse taught the wife not to push the PCA button and explained why.* Were they proper? *Yes.* Were they timely? *Yes. The student nurse did not delay. Whenever breathing or airway is threatened, nurses need to respond immediately.*

- What information was gained from the supporting roles? *The interaction between the nurse and patient's wife provided an explanation as to why the patient was receiving too much (the wife was pushing the button) and therefore we understood why the breathing was slow.* Was it realistic? *Yes! Patients and families need thorough explanations about their situation to avoid unintentionally causing problems.*

- Did the patient's condition change during the simulation? *The narrative example stopped at that point.* Why? Did the nurse recognize the change? Why or why not? *If the respiratory suppression had been worse, she could have also administered oxygen, narcan and called the physician. If calling the physician, she would have reported the level of respiratory suppression and asked for changes in the orders for the PCA so the patient would not continue to receive too much.*

- Were other interventions taken in response to the change in the patient's condition? What aspects were proper; and what might have been done differently? *(the scenario stopped at this point)*

These are the type of questions that would be covered in debriefing. In some scenarios additional concerns would include body mechanics, communication, interactions between the nurse and other caregivers, positioning in the environment, use of the chart and/or monitor and anything else that provides for your patients. You and your team members will discuss what actually occurred (or what you remember). There may be conversation about how each participant felt about the situation and responses. There would likely be some form to fill out and the opportunity for the student observers to share what they saw and were thinking.

It is not unusual for part of the scenario to require that the student nurse call the physician as part of the response to the problem (see Chapter 5). Part of the debriefing will consider this aspect of the scenario: was the physician called appropriately? Was the report complete and correct? This adds the benefit of practicing proper report in the simulation environment, too.

Each member will bring information to the discussion that you may not have thought of before this encounter. Choose to listen to your team members and be open to what they have to say. This is not a critique of what kind of person you are, but a critique of how each of the members can learn from the experience. After you and your team members have voiced your observations, the instructor will add to the conversation.

After your instructor has provided you with more information, the team may continue the discussion. Your instructor may also fast-forward the video and pause it to display aspects of the simulation. Your instructor will confirm the appropriate ideas and question the ideas that may not be on target or need redirection. Regardless, you and your team are learning important lesson about the "real world" of patient care.

The tape, or notes taken by the observers, may allow you to identify how long it took to provide specific interventions. It is difficult when you are in the middle of a situation (either real or simulated) to have an accurate idea of the passage of time. But using a tape or student observers specifically recording events makes the time frame accurate. Elapsed time is critical for so much of what we do as nurses. Together, your team and your instructor will discuss what was accomplished in a timely manner and what could have been done more effectively.

The debriefing is complete! No one got hurt, and everyone learned something!

After your debriefing is complete, your instructor may request an evaluation of the high-fidelity simulation experience. Your comments and observations are vital in developing the environment and the scenario. Your high-fidelity environments are always "under construction," and your nursing programs depend on your input for continual improvements. You are pioneers in the use of this new technology of high-fidelity simulation, and your comments will help shape nursing education of the future. Consider sharing answers to the following statements as your faculty work to improve simulation experiences:

BOX 10-1 Reflections on the simulation experience

I was really nervous about. . .

I learned the most from. . .

I did not know that the monitor provided information on. . .

Teamwork is so important because. . .

I wish I would have known. . .before the simulation.

Always remember that the patient is our focus no matter what the learning environment! Although the simulation environment does not allow practice in handling a shift, a group of patients or time management, it is excellent for practicing a specific patient situation and teamwork. This chapter has prepared you to take advantage of possible simulation opportunities your program offers as you become a nurse. Hopefully, your response to the simulation experience will be an enthusiastic question: "When can we do it again?!"

Chapter 11
Words of Wisdom

Lorene Payne, Jean Watson, Emily Stonebrook,
Ann Huntington, Cherie Howk, Mary Ellen Yonushonis,
Sheryl Cornelius, Lisa Reed, Kiera Noel Thompson,
Holly Benson, Sylvia Brown, Paige Bentley,
Lauren Shuttlesworth, Naomi Hayes, Jennifer Donwerth,
Rachel Daugherty, Maureen E. Davis, Margarita Valdes,
Dimitra Loukissa, Leslie Pafford,
and Alison Carmichael-Bishop

"Remember to stop, listen and care: the rest will follow."

—Ann Huntington

*"Nursing and caring offers a passage to the heart for this humani-
tarian gift nursing offers to mankind."*

—Dr. Jean Watson

*"Clinical is a special gift to you as a student. It's where you breathe
life into the course grade you achieved in class."*

—Alison Carmichael-Bishop

This book's conclusion is actually an exercise of inclusion. It includes advice from many nurses and recent graduates. They were asked to provide tips and advice that would help your success in nursing school clinical experiences. Their collective responses become the final chapter of this book: the WOW, the Words of Wisdom that wrap it all up.

In Chapter 1, you were invited to approach clinical rotations "from the heart." We are fortunate to have a personal reminder from Jean Watson about the importance of caring. As you continue your nursing studies, you may see more of Dr. Watson's work on the importance, and reciprocal nature, of caring. Both patient and nurse benefit when nursing care is delivered with compassion. She writes:

At this time in human history, humanity is longing for intimacy and human caring connections and authentic caring, loving relationships. Nursing and nurses are the archetype of human caring in society and are there every day offering compassionate human caring around the globe, sustaining humanity and caring for all. Nursing is an ancient and noble profession serving society and the human conditions across time. The evolved human works from the heart, not from the head alone. Nursing and caring offers a passage to the heart for this humanitarian gift nursing offers to humankind.

JEAN WATSON, PhD, RN, AHN-BC, FAAN

Distinguished Professor of Nursing, University of Colorado, Denver, College of Nursing; Founder, Watson Caring Science Institute

---

The words of a new graduate beginning her first nursing job are straight from the heart:

When I look back on nursing school clinicals, it's amazing. I can still feel the instructors looking over my shoulder. And that one time when I accidentally left the nasogastric tube unclamped remains a haunting memory. On the other hand, I can proudly say that my understanding of oncology, neuromuscular disorders, the endocrine system and electrolytes, among other things, vastly improved during my clinical experiences. However, I will never forget the way my life changed when I understood the patient.

I'm sure my nursing program was not unique in that we had all been told time and time again to study the disease processes intensely, to know our lab values like the back of our hand and to report everything to our nurses. The responsibility was so daunting. What was supposed to be a career of compassion, grace and personal touch seemed more like drills and straight memorization.

During my first medical-surgical rotation, I remember going to the hospital to prelab and look up my patient. Stressed by the amount of work that lay ahead of me in the night to come, I dropped by the patient's room on my way out to introduce myself. Mind you, this was the first patient I had taken care of in an inpatient setting. When I stepped in the room, it didn't take long before we were wrapped up in conversation, full of laughter and stories. This was the day I actually met the patient. I didn't meet the disease she had, didn't meet her lab values or her medication list. I actually met her and realized that it was not a pathology I was taking care of—it was a woman. She was full of life and also full of need. When I was doing my preparations that night, it seemed so easy because I was so interested in what she experienced with her chronic illness. I wanted to understand her and what she was coming from. I wanted to be able to confidently answer her questions the next day. This was no longer "textbook." It was real.

My eyes were opened by that experience.

If there was one thing I could tell a nursing student who is about to begin rotations, it would be to remember that it is not the disease you are caring for. It is the patient. These people are allowing you to enter and be an active part of their most intimate and challenging life experiences. The respect we must have for that is so essential. When you only have one or two patients, really getting to know them and spending time with them is so much easier.

I cannot discount the importance of knowing your material and your facts; this knowledge, along with your skills, is imperative to success. However, I don't feel that nursing school puts enough emphasis on really understanding the patient. The concept of holistic care is always mentioned, but rarely enforced. Yet this is the time to absorb the patients you care for and not only see them as a medical lesson, but as life lessons. They know when you care, and the trust that is created lets them sleep better at night. It heals them, and isn't that what is it all about?

In short, if I could tell a nursing student one thing about beginning their clinicals, it is to never forget to use your brain with your heart. Understand the patient and everything else will come. The skills will develop and the big nursing concepts will make sense. Your creativity and leadership will blossom, and your advocacy skills will have a backbone of vivacity and determination. Best of all, you will be so much more fulfilled by the path you have chosen. Nursing is a career that is deeply rooted in compassion and understanding of the person, and to me, it is this from which everything else grows.

EMILY STONEBROOK, RN

This next message of few words echoes the need to care. A student nurse working on her graduate Master's degree sends the following:

Here are my words of wisdom for any student nurse starting their initial clinical rotation: remember to stop, listen and care, the rest will follow.

ANN HUNTINGTON, RN, BSN

That reminder to "listen" is especially important. It's hard to provide what the patient needs if you don't stop and actually listen.

Here is another reminder to listen to the patient:

Dear New Clinical Student,

I have taught clinical nursing since before you were born but I can remember my first clinical experience like it was yesterday. You might be nervous or anxious about what your instructor is going to ask you, and you might feel that the written chart or computer information is overwhelming.

Pull up a chair and sit and talk with your patient. Sitting with your patient demonstrates that you are a caring nurse. You will assess more about what your patient is thinking and feeling than you will be able to assess by reading his or her chart. After sitting with your patient a while, you will know whether they are hungry, thirsty, tired, need to use the bathroom, in pain, anxious or lonely. Your patient will think that you are the best student nurse ever!

MARY ELLEN YONUSHONIS, MS, RN, CNE
The Pennsylvania State University

This faculty member reminds student nurses that students need preparation, excitement and honesty.

I believe that if nursing students come to clinical enthusiastic and excited to learn, those around them become excited about teaching them what they need to know.

I would encourage nursing students to admit when he or she does not know how to do something or are not comfortable doing a procedure. When you are asked to do something that you have not done before, it is perfectly acceptable (and encouraged) to say, "I would really appreciate being able to watch you do it this time and I will do the next one." There is always a first time to do any procedure, and students must be comfortable before they potentially put a patient in harm's way.

I do not believe any nursing staff or faculty would object to a student's honesty and interest in learning—so students must make sure that their eagerness to learn comes through when they ask to initially observe.

CHERIE HOWK, PhD, FNP-BC
Indiana State University

Here's an enthusiastic endorsement of the "hands-on" aspect of clinical rotations:

The best advice I could give to a nursing student approaching clinical is, "Jump in and see all you can see!" Volunteer for everything! The more you see the more comfortable you feel, the more comfortable you feel the more you will learn.

Those scared little students that are afraid to touch a client and are terrified to speak to a nurse or doctor are missing out on so much. So what if you are not the outgoing life of the party—fake it until you make it! If you act as though you are the most comfortable, cheery, fearless student there is, eventually you will be. This is how you gain experience.

Just as the baby bird does not learn to fly by staying under its mother's wing, your instructor cannot hold your hand all through school and then let you go at graduation expecting you to do it all on your own. You must go find experiences for yourself; ask other nurses if you can help, work weekends or summers as a Nursing Assistant (CNA) or unit secretary. When I finished school as a new graduate, I was terrified of starting an intravenous (IV) line. Once my preceptor figured this out, he made me start 16 in one day floating from unit to unit. By the end of that day, I was comfortable with IVs and love the challenge of a difficult stick to this day.

Nike had it right with all those commercials—Just Do It!

SHERYL CORNELIUS, RN, MSN
Mitchell Community College

A nurse preceptor is a staff nurse at the hospital who is a clinical expert and therefore mentors new employees of the hospital and also nursing students. Some colleges of nursing assign a student nurse to spend an entire semester with one preceptor nurse. The student always works on that unit and with that nurse expert and thus gets "on the job" training. Here are some hints for clinical success from a nurse preceptor:

Having been a nurse for 20+ years and having precepted many, many new grads and students there are two points that I like to stress. First, understand that there is never a stupid question. It is better to ask a question than to do something wrong. Secondly, seek out any and all opportunities to learn. Go with other nurses who might be doing something that you can either perform or a procedure you can learn from.

LISA REED, RN

This nursing student wants you to have patience with yourself. When you first begin clinicals, you will not be quick or polished or as efficient in your patient care.

You never forget your first patient. I had an 82-year-old man that weighed about 250 lbs. He had a left sided stroke; therefore, the right side of his body (his dominant side) was paralyzed. This man lost all of his speaking capabilities other than about three words. He was used to the way the Nursing Assistants (CNAs) took care of him.

Now here I was, a young 19-year-old student nurse. Getting him ready for breakfast took me 30–45 minutes. He was getting very frustrated with how long it was taking me and how nervous I was.

However, you need to work through it and learn through your own experiences. My advice to new students would be to really get used to helping patients who cannot move out of the bed, like changing the bed while the patient is still in it, changing a brief and using bed pans. Those skills have really helped me take care of the more difficult patients.

I feel the best way to learn is through experience, so please even if you feel embarrassed or scared, just work through it to the best of your capabilities.

KIERA THOMPSON
The Pennsylvania State University Nursing

The next two contributions come from nurses who have just completed their first year of nursing since graduation. Their words of wisdom apply even on your first clinical day.

Being a new nurse is exciting and terrifying all at once. My advice is to be cautious, yet confident in yourself and what you have learned (because somehow, all of that information is up in your brain somewhere!). Don't compare yourself to others; you're unique with your own strengths. Above all, believe in yourself, because your passion for nursing will be what makes the real difference.

Congratulations and welcome to one of the most exciting and honorable professions in the world!

HOLLY BENSON, RN

To the Student Nurse:

It seems like yesterday; I too was a student, struggling through classes, stressing about exams and wondering if I would ever make it out of nursing school! After a year of working as an RN, I have a completely different perspective. First, relax! Nursing school is stressful, but being stressed out will not help you learn.

OK, you're checked off on all your assessments and are ready to start clinical! This is exciting because it is your first step to being a real nurse. My advice to you is to seek out opportunities. Tell your preceptor and other nurses in your area to let you know if they have opportunities for skills such as placement of Foley catheter, subcutaneous injection, intramuscular injection, etc. If you are passive and do not seek out these opportunities, you may go through your entire clinical experience without learning these valuable skills. Do not be afraid to speak up.

Being an RN is so rewarding. I learn something new every day I work. There is a wealth of information awaiting you from your coworkers, patients and their families. Listen to what your patient is telling you and sometimes what they aren't. Go the extra mile for your patient. Put yourself in their shoes. What if it was you in that bed or one of your family members? How would you want to be treated?

It is my hope for you that you will enjoy your school/clinical experience, become a successful RN and achieve all that you dream of!

Best Wishes,
Sylvia Brown, RN
M. D. Anderson Cancer Center

Words from a nurse who recently graduated and is beginning her first job:

When I look back on my clinical experiences, I am struck by the importance of making the most of each day, each unit and each nurse you work with. Once you graduate from nursing school and select a specialty, you may never have the opportunity to watch the birth of a child, circulate in an operating room, or spend time with a school nurse in an elementary school. Even if you have no interest in a specific rotation, there is always something to learn.

Be prepared for clinical; be ready to ask questions and make observations. Embrace differences you see. What do these nurses do differently at this hospital? Which way would be best for your own practice? Seek out opportunities to learn and practice skills. Don't be afraid of making mistakes. Clinicals are the best time in your nursing career to make mistakes—under the watchful eye of a registered nurse who can correct and guide you.

Paige Bentley, RN, BSN

Here is a story from a nurse who recently graduated. She shares the heart of nursing.

It is said that life is comprised of milestones: birth, death and all of the wondrous events in between. There are first steps, first words, first days of school, first loves and first jobs. For every nurse, it should also be noted, there is also the life-altering experience of the first code. Four days into my internship, I experienced mine—his name was JD. The memory of this man is etched into my heart as deeply and permanently as that of anyone with whom I have shared one of life's more routine milestones. But JD and I shared something profound: I held his hand as he died, and he taught me what it means to be a nurse.

It was apparent from the first day that JD was alone in the world. While our other patients had visitors and frequent phone calls from concerned family members and friends, JD had none. His family and friends had abandoned and disowned him: he was on his own and facing a grim prognosis. It was not a surprise when he coded.

Assisting with a code is an unparalleled learning experience for a student nurse. At first, I nervously retreated to a far corner of the room, desperate not to get in anyone's way. From my vantage point, I observed with a sense of awe the meticulously choreographed chaos that was erupting around JD's bed. In spite of my desire to be inconspicuous, I was spotted by a nurse who asked if I would like to assist. As I stammered and stuttered, he instinctively recognized my panic and reminded me that practice and hands-on experience were the best way to learn.

He gently reassured me that JD's circumstances were dire, and that I most certainly would not be putting him in any greater peril than he was already facing. Freed from my anxiety, I immediately joined one of the residents who was performing chest compressions. The self-doubt and fear that had plagued me was a distant memory, and I regained my confidence.

Time seemed to stand still as everyone worked frantically to keep JD's heart beating, but in what felt like an instant, it ended. The code was called off, prompting a silent exodus of specialists from the patient's bedside. I stood there flabbergasted by the change in atmosphere. What had been a war zone only moments before instantaneously took on all of the reverence and solemnity of a funeral procession. Nothing more could be done for JD, and those who had experienced the battle between life and death many times over knew that our efforts, though colossal, were futile. The time had come to let go. Only the attending physician and I remained in the room—our eyes focused unblinking on the monitor.

I searched the attending physician's face for some sort of encouragement and found only resignation. He could do nothing more for this man in his professional capacity and, as he stood by his bedside, he willingly accepted the position that we all assume will be filled by our family members and friends.

Though the helplessness was devastating, I realized the almost sacred significance of the doctor's actions. He would remain at his patient's side until death finally took him; not merely to witness and record the particulars, but because he wasn't going to let JD die alone.

I suddenly realized exactly why fate (and some supremely talented "teachers") had conspired to put me in JD's room at such a moment. This was nursing in its purest form. I stood beside JD, choked back the enormous lump that had formed in my throat and held his hand as the waveforms became a flat line.

In that instant, I truly believe that I learned more about the field than I had from any textbook, lecture or lab: our silent vigil over a dying patient, a man nobody wanted, was the lesson of a lifetime. To be a good nurse I was going to have to make the realization that death, too, was sometimes a part of the protocol.

To this day, the thought of an unmarked, flowerless grave makes my heart ache. Whatever transpired between JD and his family was none of my business. My business was to provide him with unsurpassed care and compassion through every stage of his illness. This has been the business of nurses throughout history, and I am proud to aspire to be one of them.

LAUREN SHUTTLESWORTH, BSN, RN
Edited by ERIN RODICK
The Pennsylvania State University

More words of wisdom encouraging thought and understanding behind your nursing actions:

Your education as a student nurse improves when you ask questions. . .lots of them! Looking back, I think the best morsel of information to give would be for nursing students to keep their wits about them. Going into nursing school and clinicals can really drive your mind into some high-anxiety places. I would highly suggest to students to maintain common sense. Even though common sense is really not all that common, every little bit helps.

Maintain focus about the care that you are giving, who it is for and who will be affected by the things that you do—and the why—ask lots of questions! Why are you doing the things that you are doing, and for what purpose?

Some of the scariest nurses I have come up against are the ones who only have lists of things and boxes to check when giving medications and doing assessments. Granted, you must do these things in order, and you must have a list of objectives to accomplish, but you must also know why *you have the lists in the first place.*

Go beyond the lists, challenge yourself not just to know the list, but to know the purpose of the list. It is good to know the reasons why you are giving the care that you are giving because it allows you to understand why nursing instructors, doctors and other healthcare personnel want you to do certain things. Understanding is something that comes with time, but you can challenge yourself from the beginning to start gaining more understanding so that you can achieve better results with your work and the interactions that you have with other hospital workers, family members and patients.

NAOMI HAYES, RN

This nursing instructor offers student nurses sound advice echoed in a movie!

As I search my brain to come up with something that sums up clinical, I return to a slide I show at the start of each semester: "Improvise, adapt and overcome." It's a line Clint Eastwood tells his troops in Heartbreak Ridge (1986). I can provide my students with multitudes of information to guide them in their decision making, but unless they can be flexible in their thinking, nurses they will not be.

JENNIFER J. DONWERTH, MSN, RN, ANP-BC, GNP-BC
Faculty, Tarleton State University

In this letter to students, another instructor encourages the student to handle instructor questions during clinical rotations.

Dear Student,

You are beginning your second week of clinical rotation thinking, "I made it through the first week of clinical, perhaps I will be OK." Then you see your instructor walking toward you and your heart sinks. You know from the other students that *when she approaches you there will be a question and answer session. Now your thoughts are racing saying, "I just know she is going to ask me a question I do not have the answer for and my nursing career will be over before it begins."*

Sure enough, your instructor says, "Tell me about your patient," and you give a glowing report about your patient. The questions she asks at first are fairly easy to answer and you think, "whew." But, then she asks a question about your patient you do not know the answer to ("we have not had that in class yet, why is she asking me that?"). Could it be, your instructor is attempting to create a learning experience and is not just trying to trip you up? You see, the instructor needs to assess your knowledge base and critical thinking skills just as you need to assess your patient so you can help meet their healthcare needs.

When your clinical nursing instructor asks you a question, do not be afraid to answer. Think it through, and ask for clarification (if needed). Then take a deep breath and provide an answer as best you can, making sure you can give rationales for your answers. You survived the session with your instructor and learned something new in the process. You realize what it feels like to think like a nurse, and it really feels good.

RACHEL DAUGHERTY, MSN, RN
Assistant Professor, University of Texas Medical Branch School of Nursing

---

Postclinical conference ideas are found in these words of wisdom from an instructor.

Be creative in clinical postconference! Keep the students involved with specific objectives for each postconference. Topics could include fall risk, dysphagia, labs, perioperative, time management, diabetes and neurologic assessment.

We have the students visit the operating room (OR) once during the semester. The students report on their OR experience and discuss with other students in postconference. The students work in pairs and write a research report. One student gives a 5-minute presentation on the patient they chose to research (situation and background). The second student presents the research written by nurse researchers.

The students have been very creative in getting their fellow students involved in the patient's experience, such as research on cystic fibrosis that was presented in poster form with 10 index cards attached. Each student and the instructor chose a card and then mimicked the symptom on the card.

Some students chose interactive games and awarded prizes. They turned osteoporosis, coronary artery disease, hypertension and metabolic syndrome into games such as jeopardy, wheel of fortune, pyramid, etc.

Include speakers where possible. The director of the OR spoke about the perioperative experience. She came with all the personal protective equipment for the students to put on, pictures of the OR and discussion about staff functions.

When we covered dysphagia we actually used thicket and made liquids, which we all got a chance to mix and taste to see what the experience was like for the client before we actually fed them one-on-one in the nursing home.

Students from upper level classes came to discuss how to care for more than one patient per clinical day. The next week, the students all had their own organizational sheet for the day. Enjoy postclinical conference!

MAUREEN E. DAVIS, MSN, RN-BC
University of Texas, Austin, School of Nursing

More words of wisdom from an experienced clinical instructor and director of nursing programs. She addresses the importance of giving a good report.

When giving report, it is important that the student prioritizes information to be presented and follows a consistent pattern. This assists the nurse receiving report to organize the information and anticipate what information is going to be communicated next. Here are some important points:

- Organize the information being communicated
- Report without giving judgments or opinions
- Provide a verbal picture by communicating in an organized, concise manner

If you report well, the nurse receiving report can visualize in their mind what the client looks like. You are painting a verbal picture of your patient.

MARGARITA VALDES, MS, RN
Chief Academic Officer, Unitek College

Some clinical assignments take you to specialty areas. The following tips help you get ready for the time you may spend in a psychiatric facility.

TEN TIPS ON HOW TO SURVIVE YOUR PSYCHIATRIC CLINICAL ROTATION

"Welcome to our acute inpatient unit! We haven't lost any students recently!"

With this standard joke, the social worker of an acute psychiatric inpatient unit welcomes the already terrified nursing students for their mental health rotation.

"How old are you?" "You are hot!" "Are you married?" "You are a fat bitch!"

Psychiatric patients usually have an extraordinary ability to test trainees by asking them personal questions or making inappropriate comments. Moreover, societal stereotypes reinforce the belief that psychiatric patients are dangerous and unpredictable. Although there are very few individuals who may fall under this category, the majority of patients are human beings who are challenged with emotional and thought process difficulties. So, how can you survive as a student nurse?

1. *You are safe! Your clinical instructor will never assign you to a patient where there is even the slightest suspicion that this individual may be unpredictable. Actually, research shows that acts of violence towards staff are more common in the emergency room and acute medical units than in psychiatry.*

2. *Make peace with your feelings! Your peers feel equally unprepared, unsure and uncomfortable as you do. It is normal to feel that way in the beginning.*

3. *You are not alone! You have an entire team to help you figure things out: your clinical instructor and the entire clinical team.*

4. *There is nothing you can reasonably do or say that will make or break a patient! Learning how to communicate is one of the major challenges students are dealing with, but the only way to learn what and how to say it, is by doing it. Don't forget: your clinical instructor is right there if you would like to rehearse first.*

5. *Be open and spontaneous! There is no text to offer you an answer to every possible interaction you may have with any given patient. It is easier than you think!*

6. *Be observant! Pay attention to how staff members interact with patients, what different techniques they are using, what works, what doesn't and take the plunge!*

7. *You can always walk away from an uncomfortable interaction! If a patient is testing boundaries and you are uncomfortable setting limits, you can always excuse yourself, walk away and talk the experience over with your instructor.*

8. *Be aware of what's happening around you, even if it doesn't concern your patient. Sharing your observations with the staff can literally save the day!*

9. *Be honest! Talk about your feelings, fears and concerns with your peers and clinical instructor in postconference. You will be surprised to discover that others may have the same or similar feelings as you.*

10. *Take the journey! Be open to the new experiences! This is also a self-growth experience that will make you a wiser, more mature and better prepared person to deal with life.*

DIMITRA LOUKISSA, PhD, RN

Beginning students do not usually go to the intensive care unit because patients there have multiple problems and many organ systems involved. This nurse offers you some words of wisdom to tuck away until you go to the unit in your final semesters.

You may be overwhelmed upon first entering a patient's room. Overcome this by:

1. Assessing the patient. A thorough head-to-toe assessment is expected every 4–8 hours and ongoing focused assessments throughout the day. If you are not up to speed on assessment, review!

2. Assessing the equipment/lines/monitors. Look at each piece of equipment "attached" to the patient. Follow from the patient to the equipment or drip, you are accomplishing two things: (1) familiarizing yourself and (2) performing

safety checks. For everything attached to the patient, make sure it is working, safe, plugged in, etc.

3. IV infusions. Patients may be on multiple titrated IV medications. Follow IV lines from the patient to the infusion pump. Label the tubing close to the patient. Note the rate, drug and concentration. Do not ever assume that the previous shift calculated correctly. Recalculate all medications.

4. Providers (physicians and practitioners) frequently ask the nurse about the patient. Be aware that when you are asked, "how's Mr. Smith today?" The appropriate answer is not "fine," nor is it a lengthy story detailing every single element of care. Prioritize the patient's needs and be able to discuss them intelligently.

5. Develop a schedule for the day and keep it handy. Note all meds, labs, treatments, vital signs, assessments, lunch, etc. A well constructed and comprehensive plan can make your day much easier.

Leslie Pafford, RN, PhD, FNP-C

You have just received the collective wisdom of many nurses who would all appreciate seeing you become an excellent nurse. It is during your clinical rotations of nursing school that you have the opportunity to put all of this into practice and truly become the caregiver you would like to be.

Finally, these words of wisdom summarize clinicals perfectly!

The WOW Moment

- It's all about the patient; no one volunteers for the patient role.
- When providing care, be aware that your patient is more than just the "patient with X diagnosis." He or she has a life story and you're meeting them at a particular point in time of their journey. If your patients are abrupt, don't take it personally, but instead be compassionate and empathetic. Each patient is different and deserves a personal touch to their care.
- The best nurse is one that asks "why," knows their own limits and when in doubt asks for help.
- Nursing is more than skills/tasks (medication administration, Foley insertion, etc.); it's about listening to the patient and making a connection which may make a difference in his or her life.
- Clinical is a special gift to you as a student. It's where you breathe life into the course grade you achieved in class. If you do not take the information you learned from class and apply it in the clinical setting, it will be for naught; that letter grade will be just a "grade." It is also the first time you will see what a book can never show you: how to be a nurse. As an invited guest on the unit, be appreciative, respectful of all, be understanding and leave the unit better than when you arrived. Set goals for yourself and learn something new everyday.

- Be honest, if you do not know say, "I don't know but I will find out"; help each other and others on the unit.
- Take advantage of every learning opportunity and learn from all (administrative assistants, nurse assistant, auxiliary staff, registered nurse, practical nurses, nursing leadership and each other) you come in contact with. Learn something from everyone; you can never be taught too much.
- Although it's the clinical instructor's and preceptor's responsibility to teach, be open to learning and an active participant in the learning equation. For example, by being prepared for clinical, you will be more confident and are less likely to be intimated by your surroundings.
- And remember, always be the nurse you would want to care for your loved one and yourself.

ALISON CARMICHAEL-BISHOP, BSN, RN

There you go, student nurses. Your clinical experiences will provide the forming grounds for the type of nurse you are becoming. Embrace the learning! Care for your patients!

Welcome to Nursing!

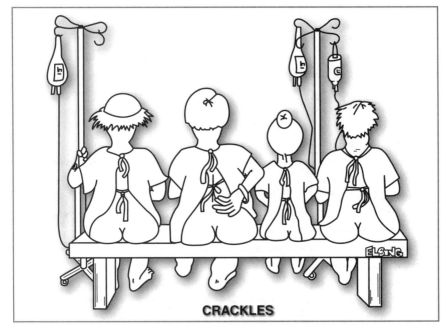

Figure 11-1   Crackles. (Courtesy of Carl Elbing. Available at http://www.nurstoon.com.)

THE END

Index